Proteomics in Laboratory Medicine

Guest Editor

EMANUEL F. PETRICOIN, PhD

CLINICS IN LABORATORY MEDICINE

www.labmed.theclinics.com

Consulting Editor
ALAN WELLS, MD, DMSc

March 2009 • Volume 29 • Number 1

SAUNDERS an imprint of ELSEVIER, Inc.

W.B. SAUNDERS COMPANY
A Division of Elsevier Inc.

1600 John F. Kennedy Boulevard ● Suite 1800 ● Philadelphia, Pennsylvania 19103-2899

http://www.theclinics.com

CLINICS IN LABORATORY MEDICINE Volume 29, Number 1

March 2009 ISSN 0272-2712, ISBN-13: 978-1-4377-0493-8, ISBN-10: 1-4377-0493-X

Editor: Joanne Husovski
Developmental Editor: Donald Mumford

Reprints. For copies of 100 or more, of articles in this publication, please contact the Commercial Reprints Department, Elsevier Inc., 360 Park Avenue South, New York, New York 10010-1710. Tel. (212) 633-3813, Fax: (212) 462-1935, E-mail: reprints@elsevier.com.

Clinics in Laboratory Medicine (ISSN 0272-2712) is published quarterly by Elsevier Inc., 360 Park Avenue South, New York, NY 10010-1710. Months of issue are March, June, September, and December. Business and Editorial offices: 1600 John F. Kennedy Blvd., Suite 1800, Philadelphia, PA 19103-2899. Customer Service Office: 6277 Sea Harbor Drive, Orlando, FL 32887-4800. Periodicals postage paid at New York, NY and additional mailing offices. Subscription prices are $204.00 per year (US individuals), $321.00 per year (US institutions), $106.00 (US students), $234.00 per year (Canadian individuals), $405.00 per year (foreign institutions), $145.00 (foreign students). Foreign air speed delivery is included in all *Clinics* subscription prices. All prices are subject to change without notice. POSTMASTER: Send address changes to *Clinics in Laboratory Medicine*, Elsevier Periodicals Customer Service 11830 Westline Industrial Drive St. Louis, MO63146. **Customer Service: 1-800-654-2452 (US). From outside of the US, call 1-314-453-7041. Fax: 1-314-453-5170. E-mail: journalscustomerservice-usa@ elsevier.com (for print support) or journalsonlinesupport-usa@elsevier.com (for online support).**

Clinics in Laboratory Medicine is covered in *EMBASE/Exerpta Medica, MEDLINE/PubMed (Index Medicus), Cinahl, Current Contents/Clinical Medicine, BIOSIS* and *ISI/BIOMED.*

Printed and bound by CPI Group (UK) Ltd, Croydon, CR0 4YY

Transferred to Digital Print 2011

Contributors

GUEST EDITOR

EMANUEL F. PETRICOIN, PhD
Co-Director, Center for Applied Proteomics and Molecular Medicine, Professor of Life Sciences, George Mason University, Manassas, Virginia

AUTHORS

AYESHA B. ALVERO, MD
Department of Obstetrics, Gynecology and Reproductive Sciences, Reproductive Immunology Unit, Yale University School of Medicine, New Haven, Connecticut

JOSIP BLONDER, MD
Laboratory of Proteomics and Analytical Technologies, SAIC-Frederick, National Cancer Institute at Frederick, Frederick, Maryland

LENORA R. BIGLER, PhD
Department of Diagnostic Sciences, University of Texas Dental Branch at Houston, Houston, Texas

SIMONA COLANTONIO, MPharm, PhD
Research Fellow, Clinical Proteomics Reference Lab, Advanced Technology Program, SAIC-Frederick, NCI-Frederick, Frederick, Maryland; Regina Elena National Cancer Institute, Rome, Italy

THOMAS P. CONRADS, PhD
Associate Professor, Department of Pharmacology & Chemical Biology, University of Pittsburgh Cancer Institute, University of Pittsburgh School of Medicine; Magee-Womens Research Institute, Pittsburgh, Pennsylvania

WILLIAM P. DUBINSKY, PhD
Department of Diagnostic Sciences, Director, CCTS Salivary Proteomics Center, University of Texas Dental Branch at Houston, Houston, Texas

VIRGINIA ESPINA, MS
Department of Molecular and Microbiology, Center for Applied Proteomics and Molecular Medicine, George Mason University, Manassas, Virginia

QIN FU, PhD
Research Associate, The Johns Hopkins Bayview Proteomics Center, Division of Cardiology, Department of Medicine, Johns Hopkins University, Baltimore, Maryland

BRIAN B. HAAB, PhD
Senior Scientific Investigator, Van Andel Research Institute, Grand Rapids, Michigan

SAM HANASH, MD, PhD
Program Head, Molecular Diagnostics Program, Division of Public Health Sciences, Fred Hutchinson Cancer Research Center, Seattle, Washington

BRIAN L. HOOD, PhD
Senior Research Scientist, Clinical Proteomics Facility, University of Pittsburgh Cancer Institute, University of Pittsburgh School of Medicine; Magee-Womens Research Institute, Pittsburgh, Pennsylvania

JON B. KLEIN, MD, PhD
Professor of Medicine and Biochemistry, James Graham Brown Endowed Chair in Proteomics, Clinical Proteomics Center, University of Louisville; Veterans Affairs Medical Center, Louisville, Kentucky

KYONGJIN KIM, MD
Department of Obstetrics, Gynecology and Reproductive Sciences, Reproductive Immunology Unit, Yale University School of Medicine, New Haven, Connecticut

LANCE A. LIOTTA, MD, PhD
University Professor, Professor of Life Sciences, Department of Molecular and Microbiology, Co-Director, Center for Applied Proteomics and Molecular Medicine, George Mason University, Manassas, Virginia

MICHAEL L. MERCHANT, PhD
Assistant Professor of Medicine, Kidney Disease Program, University of Louisville; Clinical Proteomics Center, University of Louisville, Louisville, Kentucky

GIL MOR, MD, PhD
Department of Obstetrics, Gynecology and Reproductive Sciences, Reproductive Immunology Unit, Yale University School of Medicine, New Haven, Connecticut

JI QIU, PhD
Molecular Diagnostics Program, Division of Public Health Sciences, Fred Hutchinson Cancer Research Center, Seattle, Washington

ANDREA SACCONI, DEng
Research Fellow, Clinical Proteomics Reference Lab, Advanced Technology Program, SAIC-Frederick, NCI-Frederick, Frederick, Maryland; Regina Elena National Cancer Institute, Rome, Italy

RICHARD G. SAUL, PhD, BS
Senior Scientist, Clinical Proteomics Reference Lab, Advanced Technology Program, SAIC-Frederick, NCI-Frederick, Frederick, Maryland

FLORIAN S. SCHOENHOFF, MD
Postdoctoral Research Fellow, The Johns Hopkins Bayview Proteomics Center, Division of Cardiology, Department of Medicine, Johns Hopkins University, Baltimore, Maryland; Department of Cardiovascular Surgery, University of Berne, Berne, Switzerland

NICOLAS A.S. STEWART, PhD
Research Instructor, Center for Clinical Pharmacology, Department of Medicine, University of Pittsburgh School of Medicine, Pittsburgh, Pennsylvania

CHARLES F. STRECKFUS, DDS, MA
Department of Diagnostic Sciences, Co-Director, CCTS Salivary Proteomics Center, University of Texas Dental Branch at Houston, Houston, Texas

JENNIFER E. VAN EYK, PhD
Professor of Medicine, Biological Chemistry and Biomedical Engineering, Director, The Hopkins NHLBI Proteomics Center, Director, Bayview Proteomics Group, Division of Cardiology, Department of Medicine, Johns Hopkins University, Baltimore, Maryland

TIMOTHY D. VEENSTRA, PhD
Laboratory of Proteomics and Analytical Technologies, SAIC-Frederick, National Cancer Institute at Frederick, Frederick, Maryland

IRENE VISINTIN, BA
Department of Obstetrics, Gynecology and Reproductive Sciences, Reproductive Immunology Unit, Yale University School of Medicine, New Haven, Connecticut

GORDON R. WHITELEY, PhD, MSc
Director, Clinical Proteomics Reference Lab, Advanced Technology Program, SAIC-Frederick, National Cancer Institute at Frederick, Frederick, Maryland

JULIA WULFKUHLE, PhD
Department of Molecular and Microbiology, Center for Applied Proteomics and Molecular Medicine, George Mason University, Manassas, Virginia

TINGTING YUE, BS
Research Associate, Van Andel Research Institute, Grand Rapids; Doctoral Candidate, Cell and Molecular Biology Program, Michigan State University, East Lansing, Michigan

Contents

released into the circulation allowing easy access through the blood. This article presents recent developments in autoantibody profiling with a focus on proteomic approaches and applications to lung cancer.

To overcome the significant mortality associated with ovarian cancer, a highly sensitive and specific screening test is urgently needed. CA-125 testing is used to monitor response to chemotherapy, detect recurrence, and detect late stage ovarian cancer. However, CA-125 testing, alone or in combination with ultrasonography, has not been adequate for early detection of ovarian cancer. This article discusses the authors' recent report of a novel multiplex assay that uses a panel of six serum biomarkers: leptin, prolactin, osteopontin, insulin-like growth factor II (IGF-II), macrophage inhibitory factor (MIF), and CA-125. The combination of these six proteins yielded 95.3% sensitivity and 99.4% specificity. The application of this test in the clinical context and the most appropriate population, which could benefit from the test, are discussed.

The potential of using mass spectrometry profiling as a diagnostic tool has been demonstrated for a wide variety of diseases. Various cancers and cancer-related diseases have been the focus of much of this work because of both the paucity of good diagnostic markers and the knowledge that early diagnosis is the most powerful weapon in treating cancer. The implementation of mass spectrometry as a routine diagnostic tool has proved to be difficult, however, primarily because of the stringent controls that are required for the method to be reproducible. The method is evolving as a powerful guide to the discovery of biomarkers that could, in turn, be used either individually or in an array or panel of tests for early disease detection. Using proteomic patterns to guide biomarker discovery and the possibility of deployment in the clinical laboratory environment on current instrumentation or in a hybrid technology has the possibility of being the early diagnosis tool that is needed.

Proteomic analyses by mass spectrometry are propelling the field of medical diagnostics forward at unprecedented rates because of its ability reliably to identify proteins that are at the femtomole level in concentration. These advancements have also benefited biomarker research to the point where saliva is now recognized as an excellent diagnostic medium for the detection of malignant tumors that are remote from the oral cavity. Saliva is easy to collect and may provide diagnostic information about a variety of cancers. In particular, proof-of-principle has been demonstrated for salivary biomarker research. This article reviews the literature, discusses the theories associated with saliva-based tumor diagnostics, and presents the current research focused on the use of saliva as a diagnostic medium for the detection of cancer.

Florian S. Schoenoff, Qin Fu, and Jennifer E. Van Eyk

Proteomics is fulfilling its potential and beginning to impact the diagnosis and therapy of cardiovascular disease. As de novo proteomics analysis gets more streamlined, and robust high-throughput methods are developed, more and more attention is being directed toward the field of cardiovascular serum and plasma biomarker discovery. To take cardiovascular proteomics from bench to bedside, great care must be taken to achieve reproducible results. Despite technical advances, however, the absolute number of clinical biomarkers thus far discovered by a proteomics approach is small. Although several factors contribute to this lack, one step is to build "translation teams" involving a close collaboration between researchers and clinicians.

Josip Blonder and Timothy D. Veenstra

Although proteomic technology has proved to be extremely powerful in basic research, its impact has not been as great in the clinical laboratory. The future, however, looks extremely positive because technologies, such as mass spectrometry and tissue microarrays, have continued to improve over the past several years. One of the most exciting developments, particularly in the area of mass spectrometry, is the ability to examine formalin-fixed paraffin-embedded tissue using these technologies. The almost inexhaustible supply of these tissues will enable proteomic laboratories access to clinically important specimens that will undoubtedly lead to a number of important discoveries in the near future.

Brian L Hood, Nicolas A.S. Stewart, and Thomas P. Conrads

A major goal of cancer research is elucidating the molecular events underlying carcinogenesis, with the goal of discovering better diagnostic markers and therapeutic targets. Proteomics aims to facilitate this process by applying newly developed methods and advanced analytic tools, such as mass spectrometry, for the investigation of the protein complement en masse. Proteomics is the comprehensive study of proteins and is aimed at analyzing their structure, function, modifications, expression, interactions, and localization in complex biological systems. This article reviews the state-of–the art in mass spectrometry–based approaches and their application for cancer biomarker discovery and validation.

Michael L. Merchant and Jon B. Klein

Despite significant research on many fronts, the global diabetes pandemic and its attendant complications remains complex and poorly understood. Proteomic approaches have been used to deal with these complexities through methods to increase the fractional abundance of low-abundant proteins, and to compare protein samples directly using either chemical labeling methods or label-free methods to identify and comparatively analyze proteins directly in the mass spectrometer. It is more likely that a single protein does not initiate disease progression but rather multiple vitreous-resident serum proteins likely contribute to the pathogenic mechanisms. Substantial work remains to understand better the initiation and progression of nonproliferative diabetic retinopathy, proliferative diabetic retinopathy, and diabetic macular edema in the context of why some type-1 diabetics and why many type-2 diabetics do not progress toward loss of vision and blindness.

THE CLINICS ARE NOW AVAILABLE ONLINE!

Access your subscription at:
www.theclinics.com

Preface

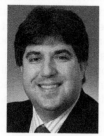

Emanuel F. Petricoin, PhD
Guest Editor

Laboratory medicine and proteomics may seem by many clinicians and research scientists, including those actively working in the field of proteomics, to be worlds apart. After all, a visitor to a typical hospital or clinical reference laboratory is not greeted with the hum of mass spectrometers and protein microarray machines busily measuring suites of clinically relevant protein analytes. Proteomics, or the comprehensive and broad-scale analysis of proteins at the "omic" or multiplexed level, however, has been a central focal point of intensive government, pharmaceutical, and academic efforts. This is because of the principal proximity of proteins as the functional control element for cellular function and disease process, and the promise that protein biomarkers bring for early detection of disease, recurrence monitoring, and tailored treatment. Although DNA is the information archive, it is the proteins that do the work of the cell. Most of the new classes of molecular inhibitors, especially for oncology, diabetes, and cardiovascular diseases, act on protein function and activity, not genes. Although pharmacogenomics has received a lot of press, proteomics may actually end up dominating the field of companion diagnostics, or theranostics: because the drug targets are most often proteins, directly measuring their presence or function provides a direct route for patient selection for response and stratification whereby the biomarker is the diagnostic and therapeutic target all-in-one (eg, c-erbB2). Many of the therapeutics themselves are proteins.

Although clinical laboratories are not yet a showcase for proteomic technologies, many clinically relevant analytes that underpin routine clinical diagnostic testing today are proteins (eg, prostate-specific antigen, C-reactive protein, CA-125, insulin growth factor-1, HER2, troponins, and so forth). The transition now occurring in clinical medicine is the need to go beyond single analyte assays to tests comprised of signatures of molecular information whereby many proteins are measured at once for a specific assay. Gone is the hope of discovering some new single protein that has all of the magical qualities of sensitivity and specificity wrapped up in one measurement. Replacing this vision is the new reality, based on rapidly evolving realization of the tremendous heterogeneity of human disease, that only through multiplexed "omic" assays will this heterogeneity be overcome by assays comprised of panels of proteins that provide the necessary positive predictive value for each indication. Proteomics is

Clin Lab Med 29 (2009) xiii–xiv
doi:10.1016/j.cll.2009.02.002
0272-2712/09/$ – see front matter © 2009 Elsevier Inc. All rights reserved.

actually an essential component of laboratory medicine today, and may represent its future.

This issue of *Clinics in Laboratory Medicine*, focusing on proteomics in laboratory medicine, represents an impressive review of the state of the field at this time. Articles focus on protein biomarker discovery and profiling for disease detection, patient-tailored therapy applications, new protein isolation-fractionation approaches along and workflows coupled to mass spectrometry, protein microarrays, and gel- and liquid-based multidimensional separation systems. Analytical considerations to evaluate the performance and fidelity of the information obtained from these efforts is also a focus of an article. Analysis of tissues, blood, and saliva are all discussed, and also reveal the flexibility and ability of proteomic technologies to mine different types of input clinical samples: essential for routine clinical implementation. The plethora of the types of protein biomarkers discussed in these articles (protein fragment isoforms, glyco-specific proteins, phosphorylated proteins, autoantibodies) are a testament to the diversity of the proteomic information archive that may represent the near-future pipeline of diagnostic, prognostic, and predictive biomarkers for the clinic.

I hope you enjoy reading this issue as much as I did. One of the greatest benefits of being invited to be an editor of an issue in The Clinics is being able to suggest content and get a glimpse into the state-of-the-art of what some brilliant scientists are doing. I wish there were 100 articles available because there are so many fantastic scientific efforts that were not able to be captured in the allotted space. The promise of proteomics is entirely translational, and the true success of these ongoing efforts can only be measured at the clinic. I believe that we are at an inflection point in these proteomic pursuits with the yardstick of success being patient benefit and not just peer-reviewed publications.

Emanuel F. Petricoin, PhD
Center for applied Proteomics and Molecular Medicine
George Mason University\10900 University Boulevard
Room 181A, Discovery Hall
Manassas, VA 20110, USA

E-mail address:
epetrico@gmu.edu

Application of Laser Microdissection and Reverse-Phase Protein Microarrays to the Molecular Profiling of Cancer Signal Pathway Networks in the Tissue Microenvironment

Virginia Espina, MS, Julia Wulfkuhle, PhD, Lance A. Liotta, MD, PhD*

KEYWORDS

- Cancer • Laser capture microdissection • Microenvironment
- Molecular profiling • Proteomics
- Reverse phase protein microarray

Genomic and proteomic research is launching the next era of cancer molecular medicine. Molecular expression profiles are revealing clues to pathogenic molecules that play a role in tumor pathogenesis and response to therapy. The next revolution is the synthesis of proteomic information into functional pathways and circuits in cells and tissues. Such synthesis must take into account the dynamic state of protein post-translational modifications and protein–protein or protein–DNA/RNA interactions, cross-talk between signal pathways, and feedback regulation within cells, between cells, and between tissues. This full set of information may be required before we can fully dissect the specific dysregulated pathways driving tumorigenesis. This higher level of functional understanding will be the basis for a true rational and individualized therapeutic design that specifically targets the molecular lesions underlying human disease. In the past, two challenges have stood in the way of routine signal pathway profiling of tumor cells in a tissue biopsy specimen. The first challenge is tissue cellular heterogeneity: tumor cells may constitute only a minority of multiple cell types in the

Department of Molecular and Microbiology, Center for Applied Proteomics and Molecular Medicine, George Mason University, 10900 University Boulevard, MS 4E3, Manassas, VA 20110, USA
* Corresponding author.
E-mail address: lliotta@gmu.edu (L.A. Liotta).

Clin Lab Med 29 (2009) 1–13
doi:10.1016/j.cll.2009.03.001
0272-2712/09/$ – see front matter © 2009 Elsevier Inc. All rights reserved.

tissue. The second challenge is the requirement for a technology that can measure the activated state of a large number of low-abundance signal pathway proteins in very small numbers of cells. Two classes of technologies were developed with the express purpose to address these challenges. The first technology, laser-capture microdissection (LCM), is used to procure specific tissue cell subpopulations under direct microscopic visualization of a standard-stained frozen or fixed tissue section on a glass microscope slide. The second class of technology is protein microarrays, which can measure hundreds of analytes in a small input sample. A particular type of protein microarray, the reverse-phase array (RPA) platform, is sensitive enough to accurately measure the small concentration of activated signal pathway molecules in microdissected tissue samples. This article explains how these two technologies, LCM and RPA, can be combined to yield molecular pathway data for the individualized therapy of the future.

MICRODISSECTION TECHNOLOGY BRINGS MOLECULAR ANALYSIS TO THE TISSUE LEVEL

Molecular analysis of pure cell populations in their native tissue environment is necessary to understand the microecology of the disease process. Accomplishing this goal is much more difficult than just grinding up a piece of tissue and applying the extracted molecules to a panel of assays. The difficulty arises because tissues are complicated, three-dimensional structures composed of large numbers of different types of interacting cell populations. The cell subpopulation of interest may constitute a tiny fraction of the total tissue volume. For example, a biopsy of breast tissue harboring a malignant tumor usually contains the following types of cell populations: (1) fat cells in the abundant adipose tissue surrounding the ducts, (2) normal epithelium and myoepithelium in the branching ducts, (3) fibroblasts and endothelial cells in the stroma and blood vessels, (4) premalignant carcinoma cells in the in situ lesions, and (5) clusters of invasive carcinoma. If the goal is to analyze the genetic changes in the premalignant cells or the malignant cells, these subpopulations are frequently located in microscopic regions occupying less than 5% of the tissue volume. Using the computer adage "garbage in, garbage out," if the extract of a complex tissue is analyzed using a sophisticated technology, the output will be severely compromised if the input material is contaminated by the wrong cells. Culturing cell populations from fresh tissue is one approach to reducing contamination; however, cultured cells may not accurately represent the molecular events taking place in the actual tissue from which they were derived. Thus, the problem of cellular heterogeneity has been a significant barrier to the molecular analysis of normal and diseased tissue. This problem is overcome by new developments in the field of laser tissue microdissection (**Fig. 1**).[1–3] LCM has been developed to provide scientists with a fast and dependable method of capturing and preserving specific cells from tissue, under direct microscopic visualization.

Given the opportunity for procuring a homogeneous population of cells from a complex tissue using LCM, the approaches to molecular analysis of pathologic processes are significantly enhanced.[1–3] The mRNA from microdissected cancer lesions has been used as the starting material to produce cDNA libraries, generate transcript microarrays, perform differential display, and discover cancer suppressor genes. Microdissection can be used to study the interactions between cellular subtypes in the organ or tissue microenvironment. Efficient coupling of LCM of serial tissue sections with multiplex molecular analysis techniques are leading to sensitive and quantitative methods to visualize three-dimensional interactions between morphologic elements of the tissue. For example, it will be possible to trace the gene expression pattern and to quantitate the protein signaling activation state along the length of a breast duct or a colonic crypt to examine the progression of neoplastic

History of Microdissection

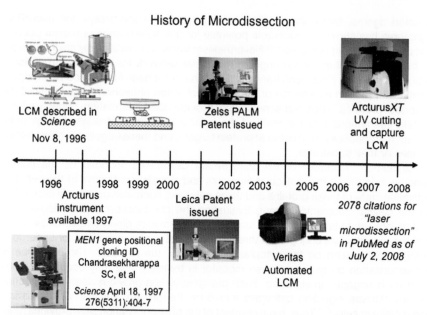

Fig. 1. The history of laser capture microdissection (LCM) as a technology for procuring pure cell populations from a stained tissue section under direct microscopic visualization. Tissues contain heterogeneous cellular populations (eg, epithelium, cancer cells, fibroblasts, endothelium, and immune cells). The diseased cellular population of interest usually makes up only a small percentage of the tissue volume. (Upper left panel) LCM directly procures the subpopulation of cells selected for study while leaving behind all of the contaminating cells. A stained section of the heterogeneous tissue is mounted on a glass microscope slide and viewed under high magnification. The experimenter selects the individual cell or cells to be studied using a joystick or by way of a computer screen. The chosen cells are lifted out of the tissue by the action of a laser pulse. The infrared laser, mounted in the optical axis of the microscope, locally expands a thermoplastic polymer to reach down and capture the cell beneath the laser pulse (*insert*). When the film is lifted from the tissue section, only the pure cells for study are excised from the heterogeneous cellular population. The DNA, RNA, and proteins of the captured cells remain intact and unperturbed. Using LCM, one to several thousand tissue cells can be captured in less than 5 minutes. Using appropriate buffers, the cellular constituents are solubilized and subjected to microanalysis methods. Proteins from all compartments of the cell can be readily procured. Protein conformation and enzymatic activity are retained if the tissues are frozen or fixed in ethanol before sectioning. The extracted proteins can be analyzed by any method that has sufficient sensitivity.

development. The end goal is the integration of molecular biology with tissue morphogenesis and pathology. LCM technology is available from a variety of vendors in several different formats.[3] The latest versions display the microscopic view of the tissue on a screen, and the operator conducts the microdissection on-screen with a computer mouse. These instruments are very reliable and relatively economical, and a current procedural terminology code is available to reimburse the pathology laboratory.

Phosphoprotein Signal Pathway Profiling

Although individualized treatments have been used in medicine for years, advances in cancer treatment have now generated a need to more precisely define and identify patients who will derive the most benefit from standard-of-care therapies and new targeted agents. Molecular profiling using gene expression arrays and microRNA signatures has shown considerable potential for the classification of patient populations by therapeutic outcome.[4–6] Nevertheless, transcript profiling, by itself, provides an incomplete picture of the ongoing molecular network for a number of clinically important reasons. First, gene transcript levels have not been found to correlate significantly with protein expression or the functional (often phosphorylated) forms of the encoded proteins. RNA transcripts also provide little information about protein–protein interactions and the state of the cellular signaling pathways. Finally, most current therapeutics are directed at protein targets, and these targets are often protein kinases or their substrates.

The human "kinome," or full complement of kinases encoded by the human genome, comprises the molecular networks and signaling pathways of the cell. The activation state of these proteins and these networks fluctuates constantly depending on the cellular microenvironment. Evaluating the combination of specific receptor protein phosphorylation sites in a tumor sample provides direct functional evidence that the receptor has changed its three-dimensional shape, dimerized, or undergone autophosphorylation on the cytoplasmic region of the receptor. The existence of phosphorylation on tyrosine kinase receptor is transient and may occur only if the receptor is engaged in signaling. Such phosphorylation provides sites of interaction for downstream signaling pathways that drive the growth, survival, differentiation, and motility of cells.[7–9] Thus, measurement of the phosphorylation sites provides functional information not obtainable by genomic or transcriptomic measurement of the receptor. Profiling kinase-driven signal pathways represents a rich source of new molecular-targeted therapeutics. Technologies that can broadly profile and assess the activity of the human kinome will be critical for the realization of patient-tailored therapy (**Fig. 2**).

Protein biomarker stability in tissue: a critical unmet need

The promise of tissue protein biomarkers to provide revolutionary diagnostic and therapeutic information will never be realized unless the problem of tissue protein biomarker instability is recognized, studied, and solved. There is a critical need to develop standardized protocols and novel technologies that can be used in the routine clinical setting for seamless collection and immediate preservation of tissue biomarker proteins, particularly those that have been posttranslationally modified, such as phosphoproteins. This critical need transcends the large research hospital environment and extends most acutely to the private practice, where most patients receive therapy. Although molecular profiling offers tremendous promise to change the practice of oncology, the fidelity of the data obtained from a diagnostic assay applied to tissue must be monitored and ensured; otherwise, a clinical decision may be based on incorrect molecular data.

Recognition that the tissue is alive and reactive following procurement

Although investigators have worried about the effects of pre-excision vascular clamping and anesthesia, a much more significant and underappreciated issue is the fact that excised tissue is alive and reacting to ex vivo stresses **Fig. 3**.

The instant a tissue biopsy specimen is removed from a patient, the cells within the tissue react and adapt to the absence of vascular perfusion, ischemia, hypoxia, acidosis, accumulation of cellular waste, absence of electrolytes, and temperature changes (see **Fig. 3**). In as little as 30 minutes post excision, drastic changes can occur in the protein signaling pathways of the biopsy tissue as the tissue remains in the operating room suite or on the pathologist's cutting board.[10] In response to

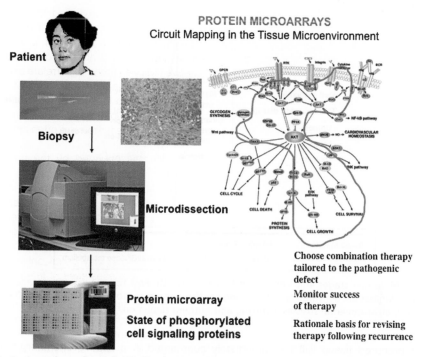

Fig. 2. A roadmap for individualized cancer therapy: following biopsy or needle aspiration and laser microdissection, signal pathway analysis is performed using protein microarrays for phosphoproteomic analysis and RNA transcript arrays. The specific signaling portrait becomes the basis of a patient-tailored therapeutic regime. Therapeutic assessment is obtained by follow-up biopsy, and the molecular portrait of signaling events is reassessed to determine whether therapeutic selection should be modified further. Reverse-phase protein microarray construction: following pathologic analysis and LCM, selected cells are lysed and printed directly onto nitrocellulose slides. Cases are printed in duplicate, with 3- to 5-point 1:2 dilution curves to ensure that the linear detection range for the antibody concentration is achieved. Controls for phospho-specific antibody specificity, such as lysates derived from cells treated with and without epidermal growth factor, are printed on every slide for quality assessment. Phosphorylation-specific reference peptides are printed in large dilution curves on the bottom of the array for comparative precise quantification of any analyte across time and experiments.

wounding cytokines, vascular hypotensive stress, hypoxia, and metabolic acidosis, it is expected that a large surge of stress-related, hypoxia-related, and wound repair–related protein signal pathway proteins and transcription factors would be induced in the tissue immediately following procurement. Over time, the levels of candidate proteomic markers (or RNA species) would be expected to widely fluctuate upward and downward over time. This fluctuation would significantly distort the molecular signature of the tissue compared with the state of the markers in vivo.[10] Moreover, the degree of ex vivo fluctuation could be significantly different between tissue types and influenced by the pathologic microenvironment. This physiologic fact must be taken into consideration as we plan to implement tissue protein biomarkers in the real world of the clinic, where the living, reacting tissue may remain in the collection basin or on the cutting board for hours. In the future, new classes of molecular fixation chemistries will be available that are just as easy to use as formalin.[10] We can envision

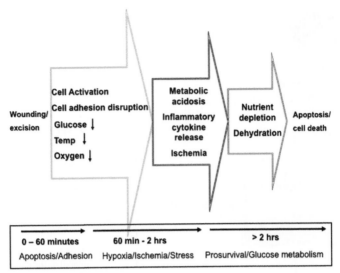

Fig. 3. Molecular stages and timeline of tissue cell death. Post tissue excision, cascades of cellular kinases are activated and deactivated as tissue reacts to wounding, ischemia, inflammation, environmental stresses, hypoxia, and nutrient depletion. Temp, temperature.

that procured tissue will be immediately submerged in a fixative chemistry that preserves phosphoproteins, proteins, RNA, DNA, and tissue morphology such that the tissue can be paraffin embedded. This process will obviate the need for dry ice transport and freezer storage for tissue specimens.

Protein Microarray Tools to Guide Patient-Tailored Therapy

Theoretically, the most efficient way to identify patients who will respond to a given therapy is to determine, before treatment initiation, which potential signaling pathways are truly activated in each patient. Ideally, this would come from analysis of tissue material taken from the patient through biopsy procurement. In general, previous traditional proteomic technologies such as two-dimensional gel electrophoresis have significant limitations when they are applied to very small tissue samples such as biopsy specimens, where only a few thousand cells may be procured. Protein microarrays represent an emerging technology that can address the limitations of previous measurement platforms and are quickly becoming powerful tools for drug discovery, biomarker identification, and signal transduction profiling of cellular material. The advantage of protein microarrays lies in their ability to provide a "map" of known cellular signaling proteins that can reflect, in general, the state of information flow through protein networks in individual specimens. Identification of critical nodes, or interactions, within the network is a potential starting point for drug development and the design of individual therapy regimens. Protein microarrays that examine protein–protein recognition events (ie, phosphorylation) in a global, high-throughput manner can be used to profile the working state of cellular signal pathways in a manner not possible with gene arrays. Protein microarrays may be used to monitor changes in protein phosphorylation over time, before and after treatment, between disease and nondisease states, and in responders versus nonresponders, allowing one to infer the activity levels of the proteins in a particular pathway in real time to tailor treatment to each patient's cellular "circuitry."[11–23]

The application of this technology to clinical molecular diagnostics is enhanced by the growing availability of high-quality antibodies that are specific for the modification or activation state of target proteins within key pathways. Antibody specificity is particularly critical, given the complex array of biologic proteins at vastly different concentrations contained in cell lysates. A cubic centimeter of biopsy tissue may contain approximately 10^9 cells, whereas a needle biopsy or cell aspirate may contain fewer than 100,000 cells. If the cell population of the specimen is heterogeneous, the final number of actual tumor cells microdissected or procured for analysis may be as low as a few thousand. Assuming that the proteins of interest and their phosphorylated counterparts exist in low abundance, the total concentration of analyte proteins in the sample is very low. Newer generations of protein microarrays with highly sensitive and specific antibodies are now able to achieve adequate levels of sensitivity for analysis of clinical specimens containing less than a few thousand cells.[11-23]

At a basic level, protein microarrays comprise a series of immobilized spots. Each spot contains a homogeneous or heterogeneous "bait" molecule. A spot on the array may display an antibody, a cell, or phage lysate; a recombinant protein or peptide; or a nucleic acid.[13,15,20] The array is queried with (1) a probe (labeled antibody or ligand) or (2) an unknown biologic sample (eg, cell lysate or serum sample) containing analytes of interest. By directly or indirectly tagging the query molecules with a signal-generating moiety, a pattern of positive and negative spots is generated. For each spot, the intensity of the signal is proportional to the quantity of applied query molecules bound to the bait molecules. An image of the spot pattern is captured, analyzed, and interpreted.

Protein microarray formats fall into two major classes, forward-phase arrays (FPAs) and RPAs, depending on whether the analytes of interest are captured from solution phase or bound to the solid phase.[15] In FPAs, capture molecules are immobilized onto the substratum and act as the bait molecule. Each spot contains one type of known immobilized protein, fractionated lysate, or other type of bait molecule. In the FPA format, each array is incubated with one test sample (eg, a cellular lysate from one treatment condition or a serum sample from disease/control patients), and multiple analytes are measured at once. A number of excellent reviews summarize recent applications, obstacles, and new advances in FPA technology[12-14] For example, arrays of human, microbial, or viral recombinant proteins can be used to screen individual serum samples from afflicted and control patients to characterize the immune response and to identify potential diagnostic markers, therapeutic targets, or radiation-regulated targets.[12-14] Antibody arrays represent another branch of FPAs that have broad applications in commercial and research settings. Examples of their use in cancer research include the identification of changes in protein levels following treatment of colon cancer cells with ionizing radiation[12] and the identification of serum protein biomarkers for bladder cancer diagnosis and outcome stratification.[23] Despite their great potential, antibody array use is currently limited by the availability of well-characterized antibodies. A second obstacle to routine use of antibody arrays surrounds detection methods for bound analyte on the array. Current options include (1) the use of specific antibodies recognizing distinct analyte epitopes from the capture antibodies (similar to a traditional sandwich-type ELISA) and (2) the direct labeling of the analytes used for probing the array—both of which present distinct technical challenges.

In contrast to the FPA format, the RPA format immobilizes an individual test sample in each array spot such that an array comprises hundreds of different patient samples or cellular lysates. Although not limited to clinical applications, the RPA format provides the opportunity to screen clinical samples that are available in limited quantities, such as biopsy specimens. Because human tissues are composed of hundreds of interacting cell populations, RPAs coupled with LCM provide a unique opportunity for discovering changes in the cellular proteome that reflect the cellular microenvironment. The RPA format is capable of extremely sensitive analyte detection, with detection levels approaching attogram amounts of a given protein and variances of less than 10%.[11,15–23] The sensitivity of detection for the RPAs is such that low-abundance phosphorylated protein isoforms can be measured from a spotted lysate representing fewer than 10 cell equivalents.[21] This level of sensitivity combined with analytic robustness is critical if the starting input material is only a few hundred cells from a biopsy specimen. Because RPA technology requires only one antibody for each analyte, it provides a facile way for broad profiling of pathways in which hundreds of phsopho-specific analytes can be measured concomitantly. Most important, the RPA has significantly higher sensitivity than bead arrays or ELISA[23] such that broad screening of molecular networks can be achieved from tissue specimens routinely procured in the physician's private office or hospital radiology center (eg, needle biopsy specimen).

Molecular Network Analysis of Human Cancer Tissues

Numerous studies illustrate the utility of RPAs for the analysis of human tissues and demonstrate the potential for the technology to contribute valuable information that can be used in therapeutic decision making. RPA technology was first described when it was used to demonstrate that prosurvival proteins and pathways are activated during prostate cancer progression.[15] Zha and colleagues[18] examined the differences in prosurvival signaling between Bcl-2–positive and Bcl-2–negative follicular lymphomas. Comparison of various prosurvival proteins by RPAs in Bcl-2–positive and Bcl-2–negative samples suggested that there are prosurvival signals independent of Bcl-2.[16] Pathway mapping of a clinical study set of childhood rhabdomyosarcoma tumors using RPAs revealed that mammalian target of rapamycin (mTOR) pathway activation correlated with response to therapy. Moreover, the functional significance of suppressing this pathway was tested in xenograft models and shown to profoundly suppress tumor growth.[19]

RPAs are also well-suited to the analysis of clinical trial material in that they can provide signaling network information that complements standard histologic analysis of patient specimens collected before, during, and after treatment. This technology is being applied to several ongoing clinical trials in a variety of cancers.

COMBINATION THERAPIES

Increasing evidence demonstrates the promise and potential of therapies that combine conventional treatments such as chemotherapy and radiotherapy with molecular-targeted therapeutics such as erlotinib (Tarceva) and trastuzumab (Herceptin) that interfere with kinase activity and protein–protein interactions in specific deregulated pathways.[24,25] Strategies that target multiple interconnected proteins within a signaling pathway, however, have not been explored to the same extent.[26,27] The view of individual therapeutic targets can be expanded to that of rational targeting of the entire deregulated molecular network extending inside and outside the cancer cell. Mathematical modeling of "network-targeted" therapeutic strategies has revealed that attenuation of downstream signals can be enhanced significantly when multiple upstream nodes or processes are inhibited with small molecule inhibitors compared with inhibition of a single upstream node. Also, inhibition of multiple nodes within a signaling cascade allows the reduction of downstream signaling to desired levels with smaller doses of the necessary targeted drugs. Although therapeutic strategies incorporating these lower dosages could lead to reduced toxicities and a broadened spectrum of available drugs, it must be recognized that testing these interacting drug modalities will necessitate clinical trials of complex design.[27]

Ultimately, therapy choice, response assessment, and therapeutic monitoring will be individualized and will reflect the subtle pre- and posttherapy changes at the proteomic level and the protein signaling cascade systems between individuals. The ability to visualize these interconnections inside and outside a cell could have a profound effect on how we view biology and could move us toward a future of personalized combinatorial molecular medicine.

Epidermal Growth Factor Receptor Phosphorylation Mapping in Lung Cancer

Targeting the epidermal growth factor receptor (EGFR) tyrosine kinase with small molecule inhibitors has received significant attention for the treatment of non–small cell lung cancer (NSCLC). Gefitinib (Iressa) and erlotinib have shown significant clinical benefit in specific subsets of lung cancer patients.[28–30] Promising phase I trial results with gefitinib demonstrated that the drug decreased levels of activated EGFR and mitogen-activated protein kinase in posttreatment skin biopsy specimens, indicating that the intended target was being inhibited.[30–33] Subsequent international phase II trials in patients who had progressive NSCLC (Iressa Dose Evaluation in Advanced Lung Cancer trial IDEAL I and II), showed 18.4% and 10% response rates, respectively, based on radiographic assessment.[31,32] These observations led to exploration of clinical factors that distinguish the small minority of patients who respond durably to these EGFR tyrosine kinase inhibitors. Further analysis of this small subset led to the sequencing and identification of EGFR mutations that are associated with sensitivity to these drugs.[29,30] The presence of EGFR mutations correlates remarkably well with the identified correlative clinical parameters.

To date, the differences in signaling between wild-type and mutant EGFRs are poorly understood. It is not clear whether the various EGFR mutations possess distinct signaling, altered sensitivities to EGFR inhibitors, or both. Moreover, there is a subset of patients who do not have EGFR mutations (ie, mutations mainly in exons 19 and 21) that respond to EGFR inhibitors.[30] The EGFR signaling network can be activated in a number of ways: mutation of the receptor, overexpression of the receptor, and mutation of downstream kinases such as phosphatidylinositol 3-kinase (PI3K), to name a few. This multi-receptor/protein activation suggests that mutation analysis alone should not serve as the sole criteria for identification and treatment selection and that further studies incorporating proteomic profiling of tissue may be beneficial in identifying additional patients who will benefit from EGFR tyrosine kinase inhibitor treatment. Proteomic profiling of EGFR-related signaling activity in preclinical and in vitro experiments and in clinical specimens could provide useful information for characterizing drug responses.[21] RPA technology is well suited to assess the signaling differences between mutant and wild-type cells, and these studies are currently underway.

The authors quantitatively profiled the phosphorylation and abundance of signal pathway proteins relevant to the EGFR within LCM untreated, human NSCLC (n = 25) of known EGFR mutation status.[21] The authors measured six phosphorylation sites on EGFR to evaluate whether EFGR mutation status in vivo was associated with the coordinated phosphorylation of specific multiple phosphorylation sites on the EGFR and downstream proteins. RPA quantitation of NSCLC revealed simultaneous up-regulation of EGFR residues Y1148 and Y1068, and down-regulation of EGFR Y1045, Her2 Y1248, IRS-1 ser612, and Smad Ser465/467, across all types of mutated

EGFR patient samples compared with wild-type. To explore which subset of these correlations was influenced by the microenvironment versus an intrinsic phenotype of the EGFR mutants, the authors profiled the time course of 112 cellular signal proteins for epidermal growth factor ligand–stimulated NSCLC mutant and wild-type cultured cell lines. EGFR mutant cell lines displayed a similar pattern of EGFR Y1148, Y1068 and Y1045, and Her2 Y1248 phosphorylation to that found in tissue. Persistence of phosphorylation for protein kinase B (AKT) ser473 following ligand stimulation was found for the mutant. In contrast to the tissue, the cell lines did not exhibit the association of EGFR phosphorylation with insulin receptor substrate (IRS-1) ser 612 or the reduction in Smad2 ser465/467. The authors hypothesized that the tissue microenvironment influences signaling through insulin-like growth factor and transforming growth factor β, thus explaining this difference. These data suggest that a higher proportion of the EGFR mutant carcinoma cells may exhibit activation of the PI3K/AKT/mTOR pathway through Y1148 and Y1068 and suppression of IRS-1ser612, altered heterodimerization with erythroblastic leukemia viral oncogene homolog 2 (ErbB2), reduced response to transforming growth factor β suppression, and reduced ubiquitination/degradation of the EGFR through EGFR Y1045, thus providing a survival advantage.

Multiple Phosphorylation Sites on the Epidermal Growth Factor Receptor are Altered in the Epidermal Growth Factor Receptor Mutant Carcinomas

More than 13 distinct phosphorylation sites exist on the EGFR.[34] The specific type of phosphorylation, the simultaneous phosphorylation of multiple sites, and the time course of the phosphorylation can all influence the proteins that dock with the cytoplasmic tail of the receptor.[35] In this way, the timing and pattern of phosphorylation events can regulate the downstream pathway interconnections emanating from the hetero- or homodimerization of the EGFR with other cell surface receptors in response to autocrine or paracrine ligands. The autophosphorylation sites inside the intracellular tail often serve as docking sites for a range of proteins, and initiate cascades of separate and functionally distinct downstream signal pathways.[34,35] Sequence mutations in the cytoplasmic tail are known to affect phosphorylation and the resultant intracellular protein binding.[35] Previous studies of posttranslational modifications of EGFR have indicated that phosphorylation events are transient, rapidly fluctuating over time.[34] Indeed, the temporal fluctuation of EGFR is thought to be the major mechanism by which a small family of receptors can influence a wide diversity of cellular functions such as regulation, differentiation, and even apoptosis.[35] These spatial and temporal fluctuations of EGFR phosphorylation could be causal determinants in diseases such as cancer. Unsupervised hierarchic clustering revealed simultaneous up-regulation of EGFR residues Y1148 and Y1068 and down-regulation of Her2 Y1248 and EGFR Y1045 in the mutated EGFR patient samples compared with wild-type.[21] Based on what is known from cell line studies of the wild-type receptor, these phosphorylation sites play a role in the docking of the receptor with downstream signal pathways in the PI3K/AKT/mTOR, the Shc (Src holomologs and collagen), and the MEK/ERK (Mitogen activated protein kinase/Extracellular receptor kinase) networks. In theory, stimulated EGFR could activate a wide variety of downstream signaling pathways. The limited number of downstream hyperphosphorylated, activated proteins is in keeping with the expected docking partners for the EGFR phosphorylation sites that are simultaneously up-regulated in the mutant. Thus, an elevated level of phosphorylation at AKT ser473, ERK T202/Y204, SHC Y317, Fox01 Forkhead T24, Elongation Binding Protein 1 Ser65, ErbB2, Y1248, Endothelial Nitric Oxide Synthase Ser1177, Src Y527, Src Y416, Bcl-2 Ser70, mTOR Ser2481, Platelet Derived Growth

Factor Receptor Beta Y716, Elongation Initiation Factor 4G Ser1108, or Focal Adhesion Kinase Y576 suggests that the signaling pathways associated with these EGFR docking proteins are activated. This activation would drive oncogenic cell proliferation/survival, cell migration/invasion, and cell differentiation.

SUMMARY

Instead of subjective immunohistochemistry scoring of selected protein analytes such as EGFR and ErbB2, future pathology reports can be envisioned to include a complete quantitative phosphoproteomic portrait of the functional state of many relevant specific downstream end points and entire classes of signaling pathways. This new class of information will serve as a guide for therapeutic decision making and prognosis. Molecular profiling of the proteins and signaling pathways active within the tumor microenvironment hold great promise in effective selection of therapeutic targets in the stroma and the vasculature. For many of the more common sporadic cancers, there is significant heterogeneity in cell signaling, tissue behavior, and susceptibility to current therapies. Cataloging of abnormal signaling pathways for large numbers of specimens will provide the population data necessary for a rationally based formulation of combination therapy that has the potential to be more effective than monotherapy. The promise of proteomic-based profiling, as distinct from gene transcript profiling alone, is that the resulting prognostic signatures are derived from drug targets (eg, activated kinases) and not from genes, so the pathway analysis provides a direction for therapeutic mitigation. Thus, phosphoproteomic pathway analysis becomes a diagnostic/prognostic signature and a guide to therapeutic intervention.

REFERENCES

1. Emmert-Buck MR, Bonner RF, Smith PD, et al. Laser capture microdissection. Science 1996;274:998–1001.
2. Ma XJ, Salunga R, Tuggle JT, et al. Gene expression profiles of human breast cancer progression. Proc Natl Acad Sci U S A 2003;100:5974–9.
3. Espina V, Wulfkuhle JD, Calvert VS, et al. Laser capture microdissection. Nat Protoc 2006;1(2):586–603.
4. van de Vijver MJ, He YD, van't Veer LJ, et al. A gene-expression signature as a predictor of survival in breast cancer. N Engl J Med 2002;347:1999–2009.
5. Bullinger L, Döhner K, Bair E, et al. Use of gene-expression profiling to identify prognostic subclasses in adult acute myeloid leukemia. N Engl J Med 2004; 350:1605–16.
6. Calin GA, Croce CM. MicroRNA signatures in human cancers. Nat Rev Cancer 2006;6(11):857–66.
7. Petricoin EF III, Bichsel VE, Calvert VS, et al. Mapping molecular networks using proteomics: a vision for patient-tailored combination therapy. J Clin Oncol 2005; 23:3614–21.
8. Yokoyama N, Malbon CC. Phosphoprotein phosphatase-2A docks to dishevelled and counterregulates Wnt3a/β-catenin signaling. Published online 2007 October 25. J Mol Signal 2007;2:12. doi:10.1186/1750-2187-2-12.
9. Bain Jenny, Plater L, Elliott M, et al. The selectivity of protein kinase inhibitors: a further update. Biochem J 2007;408(Pt 3):297–315.
10. Espina V, Edmiston KH, Heiby M, et al. A portrait of tissue phosphoprotein stability in the clinical tissue procurement process. Mol Cell Proteomics 2008; 7(10):1998–2018.

11. Wulfkuhle JD, Speer R, Pierobon M, et al. Multiplexed cell signaling analysis of human breast cancer applications for personalized therapy. J Proteome Res 2008;7:1508–17.
12. Sreekumar A, Nyati MK, Varambally S, et al. Profiling of cancer cells using protein microarrays: discovery of novel radiation-regulated proteins. Cancer Res 2001; 61:7585–93.
13. LaBaer J, Ramachandran N. Protein microarrays as tools for functional proteomics. Curr Opin Chem Biol 2005;9:14–9.
14. Robinson WH. Antigen arrays for antibody profiling. Curr Opin Chem Biol 2006; 10:67–72.
15. Paweletz CP, Charboneau L, Bichsel VE, et al. Reverse phase protein microarrays which capture disease progression show activation of pro-survival pathways at the cancer invasion front. Oncogene 2001;20:1981–9.
16. Gulmann C, Espina V, Petricoin EF III, et al. Proteomic analysis of apoptotic pathways reveals prognostic factors in follicular lymphoma. Clin Cancer Res 2005;11: 5847–55.
17. Sheehan KM, Calvert VS, Kay KW, et al. Use of reverse-phase protein microarrays and reference standard development for molecular network analysis of metastatic ovarian carcinoma. Mol Cell Proteomics 2005;4:346–55.
18. Zha H, Raffeld M, Charboneau L, et al. Similarities of prosurvival signals in Bcl-2-positive and Bcl-2-negative follicular lymphomas identified by reverse phase protein microarray. Lab Invest 2004;84:235–44.
19. Petricoin EF III, Espina V, Araujo RP, et al. Phosphoprotein pathway mapping: akt/mammalian target of rapamycin activation is negatively associated with childhood rhabdomyosarcoma survival. Cancer Res 2007;67(7):3431–40.
20. Wulfkuhle JD, Edmiston KH, Liotta LA, et al. Technology insight: pharmacoproteomics for cancer-promises of patient-tailored medicine using protein microarrays. Nat Clin Pract Oncol 2006;3:256–68.
21. VanMeter AJ, Rodriguez AS, Bowman ED, et al. Laser capture microdissection and protein microarray analysis of human non-small cell lung cancer: differential epidermal growth factor receptor (EGFR) phosphorylation events associated with mutated EGFR compared with wild type. Mol Cell Proteomics 2008;7(10): 1902–24.
22. Nishizuka S, Charboneau L, Young L, et al. Proteomic profiling of the NCI-60 cancer cell lines using new high-density reverse-phase lysate microarrays. Proc Natl Acad Sci U S A 2003;100:14229–34.
23. Grote T, Siwak DR, Fritsche HA, et al. Validation of reverse phase protein array for practical screening of potential biomarkers in serum and plasma: accurate detection of CA19-9 levels in pancreatic cancer. Proteomics 2008;8(15):3051–60.
24. Araujo RP, Petricoin EF, Liotta LA. A mathematical model of combination therapy using the EGFR signaling network. Biosystems 2005;80:57–69.
25. Araujo RP, Doran C, Liotta LA, et al. Network-targeted combination therapy: a new concept in cancer treatment. Drug Discov Today 2004;1:425–33.
26. Arteaga CL, Baselga J. Clinical trial design and end points for epidermal growth factor receptor-targeted therapies: implications for drug development and practice. Clin Cancer Res 2003;9:1579–89.
27. Gasparini G, Gion M. Molecular-targeted anticancer therapy: challenges related to study design and choice of proper endpoints. Cancer J Sci Am 2000;6:117–31.
28. Giaccone G. Epidermal growth factor receptor inhibitors in the treatment of non-small-cell lung cancer. J Clin Oncol 2005;23:3235–42.

29. Lynch TJ, Bell DW, Sordella R, et al. Activating mutations in the epidermal growth factor receptor underlying responsiveness of non-small-cell lung cancer to gefitinib. N Engl J Med 2004;350:2129–39.
30. Paez JG, Janne PA, Lee JC, et al. EGFR mutations in lung cancer: correlation with clinical response to gefitinib therapy. Science 2004;304:1497–500.
31. Fukuoka M, Yano S, Giaccone G, et al. Multi-institutional randomized phase II trial of gefitinib for previously treated patients with advanced non-small-cell lung cancer. J Clin Oncol 2003;21:2237–46.
32. Kris MG, Natale RB, Herbst RS, et al. Efficacy of gefitinib, an inhibitor of the epidermal growth factor receptor tyrosine kinase, in symptomatic patients with non-small cell lung cancer. A randomized trial. JAMA 2003;290:2149–58.
33. Wu SL, Kim J, Bandle RW, et al. Dynamic profiling of the post-translational modifications and interaction partners of epidermal growth factor receptor signaling after stimulation by epidermal growth factor using Extended Range Proteomic Analysis (ERPA). Mol Cell Proteomics 2006;5:1610–27.
34. Oksvold MP, Thien CB, Widerberg J, et al. Serine mutations that abrogate ligand-induced ubiquitination and internalization of the EGF receptor do not affect c-Cbl association with the receptor. Oncogene 2003;22:8509–18.
35. Hynes NE, Lane HA. ERBB receptors and cancer: the complexity of targeted inhibitors. Nat Rev Cancer 2005;5:341–54.

Microarrays in Glycoproteomics Research

Tingting Yue, BS[a,b], Brian B. Haab, PhD[a,*]

KEYWORDS

- Glycobiology • Glycoproteomics • Glycan microarrays
- Lectin microarrays • Antibody microarrays

The importance of carbohydrate posttranslational modifications on proteins has become increasingly clear over many decades of advances in the understanding of glycobiology. It is now widely appreciated that the carbohydrate side chains play critical roles in the structure and function of most cell surface and secreted proteins. These roles include the guiding of proper protein folding, the maintenance of protein conformation, mediating receptor-ligand and protein-protein interactions, providing biophysical polarity or hydrophilicity, and guiding immune recognition.[1] Abnormal glycosylation also is associated with a variety of inherited and sporadic diseases,[2,3] testifying to the necessity of proper glycosylation for the maintenance of health. Furthermore, glycosylation has been found to be an integral part of the proper functioning of every organism in nature. Given this broad importance of glycobiology, the field has increasing importance in applied research in biotechnology and biomedicine. For example, treatment strategies based on interfering with glycan-mediated processes or targeting cancer glycans are under development,[4] and blood-based diagnostic tests using glycan detection may be possible.[2]

Protein glycosylation refers to the chains of monosaccharide building blocks that are covalently linked to particular amino acid residues (usually serine, threonine, or asparagine residues). The monosaccharides are often five- or six-carbon cyclic structures with various modifications and isometries. Glycosidic bonds join the monosaccharides at any of the carbons with either an alpha or a beta linkage (referring to the stereoisometry of the linkage at a chiral carbon) and in a linear or branched fashion. This variety in the components and the linkages results in a huge diversity of structures that can be formed. In reality, although great diversity indeed is observed in each

This work is supported by the NCI (grant R33 CA122890) and the Van Andel Institute.
[a] Van Andel Research Institute, 333 Bostwick NE, Grand Rapids, MI 49503, USA
[b] Cell and Molecular Biology Program, Michigan State University, East Lansing, MI 48824, USA
* Corresponding author.
E-mail address: brian.haab@vai.org (B.B. Haab).

organism, particular motifs and structural themes are prevalent, bringing some order to the complexity.

The study of carbohydrate biology has been viewed as daunting by many researchers because of the heavy chemistry emphasis and perceived difficulty in the traditional analytical methods. Indeed, historic glycobiology has focused primarily on carbohydrate chemistry and involved techniques not typically included in the education of biologists. The development of modern biologic methods provided new ways of studying glycobiology, however, resulting in huge advances in the understanding of the genetic and biochemical basis of glycan synthesis and the molecular and cellular biology of glycans. The new tools for studying glycobiology make the field more accessible and useful to a broader base of researchers. These new tools include glycan-binding antibodies and proteins, genetically modified cells and organisms, gene expression profiling of glycan-related genes, and advanced chromatographic and mass-spectrometry analysis of glycan structures.

Another set of tools that is advancing glycobiology is built on the microarray platform. Microarray methods analyzing RNA and DNA transformed gene expression and genetic research following their introduction in the early 1990s.[5] The usefulness of the microarray platform lies in its multiplexing capability (enabling the acquisition of many data points in parallel) and its miniaturization (resulting in very small consumption of reagents and samples). These benefits were recognized by researchers studying other molecule types, including proteins, antibodies, lipids, and glycans, but microarrays for such studies developed more slowly because of increased technical difficulty. Currently, microarrays for studying all types of molecules are becoming established and broadly applied.

This article deals with the application of microarray formats to the study of glycoproteins and glycans. The technology and applications of three different types of microarrays developed for glycoproteomics research are surveyed: (1) glycan microarrays, (2) lectin microarrays, and (3) antibody-lectin sandwich microarrays (**Fig. 1**). Each format is used in distinct and complementary types of experiments and has facilitated advances in glycobiology research. The article focuses on glycans and proteins and does not cover DNA arrays, such as the Glyco-gene DNA chip (provided by the Consortium for Functional Glycomics) for profiling the expression of genes involved in the glycosylation machinery.

GLYCAN MICROARRAYS

A major goal in glycobiology research is to probe and characterize interactions between glycans and various types of glycan-binding proteins. Conventional methods for such studies are not suitable for the profiling of many different glycans (glycomics studies). For example, the glycan-binding specificities of lectins have been effectively probed by determining the elution profiles of various glycans in affinity chromatography,[6] but these experiments require a significant amount of glycan material per test with each glycan tested sequentially. Likewise, enzymatic studies on glycans can only be performed on a single glycan per assay and require significant material.

The glycan microarray addresses these limitations by enabling binding analyses to many different carbohydrate structures in small sample volumes and with minimal consumption of the reagents. The low consumption of the carbohydrate structures is particularly important because of the difficulty and time required to synthesize or isolate those structures. An overview is presented next of the types of carbohydrate microarrays that have been produced, follow by a review of the applications of carbohydrate microarrays.

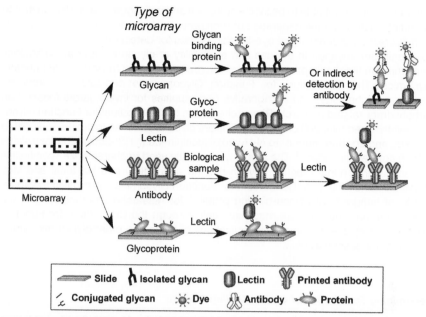

Fig. 1. Microarray formats for glycoproteomics research. The types of microarrays depicted are glycan arrays, lectin arrays, antibody-lectin sandwich arrays, and glycoprotein arrays. A detection strategy using a fluorescent dye is depicted, although other detection methods could be used, such as surface-plasmon resonance or chemiluminescence. Glycoprotein arrays, involving the isolation of glycoproteins from biologic samples using chromatographic methods, followed by the probing by lectins of the glycans microarrayed proteins,[64,65] are not discussed in the text but are depicted here for completeness.

Technologic Overview

Several different demonstrations of carbohydrate microarrays appeared in 2002 with a variety of fabrication techniques.[7,8] Houseman and Mrksich[9] used covalent attachment of carbohydrate-cyclopentadiene conjugates to self-assembled monolayers on gold surfaces to create monosaccharide arrays, and these chips were used to test interactions with selected lectins and enzymes. Monosaccharide and disaccharide chips were created by Park and Shin[10] using the covalent attachment of maleimide-linked carbohydrates to thiol-derivatized slides. Fazio and colleagues[11] attached oligosaccharides to hydrocarbon chains, which were then attached in a noncovalent fashion to the bottoms of wells of polystyrene microtiter plates. These oligosaccharides were probed with lectins and also were modified directly in the plate using glycosyltransferases. Wang and colleagues[12] used noncovalent attachment to create glycan microarrays, by spotting carbohydrate-containing macromolecules onto nitrocellulose-coated glass slides. A wide variety of microbial antigens were probed with anticarbohydrate antibodies. Fukui and colleagues[13] also used a nitrocellulose surface, onto which they spotted lipid-linked oligosaccharide probes generated from glycoproteins and polysaccharides. Noncovalent attachment also was used by Willats and coworkers,[14] in which complex polysaccharides, proteoglycans, and neoglycoproteins were spotted onto oxidized polystyrene, followed by probing with antiglycan antibodies. Several of these applications show the value of oligosaccharides derived from biologic sources, which represent complex, biologically relevant structures that are not able to be synthesized. Xia and colleagues[15] also demonstrated a practical method for the generation of such probes. These demonstrations primarily used fluorescence scanning of dye-labeled probes for detection.

A significant advance in the use and availability of glycan microarray technology came through the development of glycan microarrays by the Consortium for Function Glycomics. The Consortium for Function Glycomics is dedicated to providing resources, technology, and collaborative opportunities for investigators focused on carbohydrate-related research. Researchers from the Consortium for Function Glycomics synthesized over 200 biologically relevant glycans attached to amine-conjugated spacers, and spotted them onto N-Hydroxysuccinimide (NHS)-activated glass slides to form covalent linkages.[16] The arrays were initially used to characterize specificities of plant lectins, human lectins, glycan-binding antibodies, and bacterial and viral proteins.[16] Since then, the Consortium for Function Glycomics has profiled the specificities of hundreds of glycan-binding proteins for researchers participating in the consortium, and the data are made available through the Consortium for Function Glycomics Web site. Some of the applications of these and other glycan microarray platforms are described next.

Determining Specificities of Glycan-Binding Proteins

The most widely used application of glycan microarrays is to characterize the specificities of glycan-binding proteins and antibodies. An important class of molecules for which glycan-binding specificity has been studied is lectins, which are nonenzymatic, glycan-binding proteins found in all types of organisms. Lectins play roles in diverse processes, such as cell migration, immune recognition, and angiogenesis,[17] and information about lectin-binding specificities gives important clues about function. In addition, the characterization of lectin specificity is helpful for its use as an analytical reagent.

Manimala and colleagues[18] developed a glycan microarray containing 54 conjugated glycans, ranging from basic monosaccharides to more complicated cancer-associated glycan motifs, to obtain the binding profiles of 24 lectins. Glycan microarray slides were incubated with biotinylated lectins in serial dilutions and probed with streptavidin-horseradish peroxidase. The authors identified specificities that were not previously observed because of the lack of practical approaches for screening that number of interactions. For example, a similar study using the conventional ELISA method requires the use of over 100-fold more sample.

Glycan microarrays also have been useful to characterize the specificities of monoclonal antibodies raised against carbohydrates. Microarrays containing 80 different carbohydrates were used by Manimala and coworkers[19] to study the specificities of 27 different antiglycan antibodies, which showed that most antibodies bound other glycans in addition to their nominal targets. This finding may reflect the difficulty in generating truly specific antiglycan antibodies. The same group also showed that antibodies raised against the Tn antigen (GalNAca1-O-Ser/Thr), an important epitope in cancer and microbiology, also reacted with the blood group A structure (a related glycan), which has implications for diagnostics using antiglycan antibodies.[20] In related applications, the glycan-binding specificities of antibodies raised against the cell wall polymers from the plant Arabidopsis thaliana were characterized using arrays containing 50 cell wall glycans,[21] and specialized microarrays were designed to characterize the specificities of monoclonal antibodies targeting the Globo H hexasaccharide found on cell surfaces from breast, prostate, and ovarian cancers.[22]

Antiglycan Immune Responses Characterized Using Glycan Arrays

Certain glycan structures can elicit an immune response if the structures are not normally presented to the host immune system. Indeed, the blood group glycan structures of the ABO system elicit antibodies against structures not found in the host, which can lead to the agglutination of red blood cells from unmatched blood. Antiglycan antibodies also can be generated in immune responses against pathogens and cancer. The glycan array provides a powerful tool for probing for antiglycan antibodies and for determining their specificities. In the work of Lawrie and colleagues,[23] a glycan microarray containing 37 covalently bound glycans was used to identify carbohydrates that trigger humoral immune responses in classical Hodgkin's lymphoma patients. Total IgG and IgM from groups of patient and age- and gender-matched control individuals were purified, pooled within the same diagnostic states, and applied to individual arrays. Biotin-conjugated anti–human IgG or IgM antibodies, followed by dye-labeled streptavidin and fluorescence scanning, were used to detect antiglycan antibodies. Antibodies against five carbohydrates, including the T and Tn antigens (Galβ1,3GalNAcα- and GalNAcα-, respectively) were identified from classical Hodgkin's lymphoma patients and became targets for further investigation.

In another cancer-related study, glycan microarrays were used by Wang and colleagues[24] to show that breast cancer patients have an increased level of antibodies targeting a glycan structure called Globo H, which is found on the surfaces of breast cancer cells. Globo H and its truncated analogs were robotically spotted at various concentration onto NHS-coated glass slides for covalent attachment, and bound antibodies were detected by Cy3-labeled anti-IgG secondary antibodies. The detection of anti–Globo H antibodies may be useful for breast cancer diagnostics.

Antibodies against bacterial pathogens also were detected using carbohydrate arrays. Arrays containing glycans from anthrax toxin (*Bacillus anthracis*) were generated to characterize antibodies from rabbits that had been infected with anthrax.[25] Antibodies were found that reacted with a prominent tetrasaccharide specifically found on the spore surface, which confirms this structure as an important immunologic target. A carbohydrate microarray containing oligosaccharides specific for different versions of *Salmonella enterica* was used to identify glycan-reactive antibodies and to confirm the presence of strain subgroups in patients suffering from salmonellosis.[26] This method might be useful for rapid diagnosis or for epidemiologic or vaccine studies.

Microbiology Applications

Glycans play important roles in the recognition and attachment to host sites by microbial pathogens. In most cases the nature of the glycan attachment sites is not known. Glycan microarrays have been useful for studying that question. Stevens and colleagues[27] used glycan microarrays to investigate the host specificity of influenza viruses. Glycans with different carbohydrate components or glycosidic linkages printed in the microarray were incubated with recombinant hemagglutinins from membranes of various influenza virus strains or hybridized directly with whole virus. Different virus strains were found to have distinct preferences of binding to particular glycosidic linkage types. Profiling of strain-specific glycoprotein binding specificity from various virus strains using glycan microarray could provide crucial information in understanding virus adaptation and species barriers, which may be useful for preventing human infection.

Disney and Seeberger[28] used glycan microarrays containing five different monosaccharides to detect pathogens and test for their antibiotic susceptibility. Microarray slides were hybridized with *Escherichia coli* cells that had been labeled with a nucleic acid staining dye. After washing away unbound bacteria, slides were scanned to detect fluorescence, indicating the glycan-bacteria binding. Mutant strains with altered carbohydrate binding patterns could be detected from this assay. The authors proposed that a carbohydrate-binding "fingerprint" identified using this glycan microarray can be used to determine the types of bacteria present within a complex mixture. Because this is a nondestructive method, bacteria captured on the arrays can further be harvested and tested for antibacterial susceptibility, which is not possible using traditional destructive methods, such as those requiring polymerase chain reaction.

Enzymatic Studies

Another important application of glycan microarrays is to evaluate the specificities and activities of sugar-processing enzymes, such as transferases used for the addition of carbohydrate units.[29–31] Increased knowledge about glycosyltransferases and glycosidases would lead to a better understanding of how certain glycan chains are produced and how to use these enzymes for the synthesis of carbohydrates. Several groups have demonstrated the modification of sugars immobilized in arrays. In the work of Park and Shin,[30] the treatment of glycan arrays with UDP-Gal and β-1,4-galactosyltransferase resulted in the conversion of *N*-acetylglucosamine (GlcNAc) to lactosamine only in the absence of fucose on the GlcNAc, providing valuable information about the enzyme specificity. In another experiment from the same group, the authors successfully synthesized Sialyl Le^x (NeuNAcα2,3Galβ1,4(Fucα1,3)GlcNAc) from arrayed GlcNAc by the addition of a series of glycotransferase and sugar units.[29] Their work showed the efficiency and potential of using glycan microarray to characterize carbohydrate-processing enzymes and the possibility of enzymatic transformation from simple glycans to complex carbohydrates directly on the array. In more recent work, the acceptor specificities of multiple sialyltransferases were compared, showing differences in substrates between human and rat sialyltransferases.[31]

LECTIN MICROARRAYS

Lectin microarrays also take advantage of the low-volume and multiplexing capabilities of microarrays, but provide complementary information to glycan microarrays. Lectins were first recognized by their ability to agglutinate red blood cells,[32] and later the term "lectin" was adopted when it was realized that there existed a class of carbohydrate-binding proteins.[32] Although lectins were originally isolated from plants, they were later found ubiquitously in nature.[33] Lectins originally were classified according to their glycan-binding specificities, but they are now more consistently grouped according to sequence and structural motifs.[34]

Plant lectins have become extremely valuable analytical tools for the detection of particular carbohydrate structures. As affinity reagents, lectins can detect glycans with high reproducibility and in a variety of formats, and provide a good alternative to other glycan detection methods involving enzymatic digestion, chromatography, or mass spectrometry, which have low reproducibility and low throughput. The specificity of detecting particular glycans depends on the lectin used; some are highly specific, and others have broad specificities. Lectin detection can have good sensitivity because of multivalent binding, resulting from either a multisubunit or multiple carbohydrate-binding sites within a single polypeptide.[1]

Lectins have long been used for detection and purification of glycans in various research fields.[35] Lectins have been used extensively in immunohistochemistry (eg, in studies to examine the tissue distribution in pancreatic tumors of certain blood-group carbohydrates).[36,37] Lectins also have been used in immunoaffinity electrophoresis and blotting methods (eg, to identify cancer-associated glycan variants on the serum proteins α-fetoprotein,[38] haptoglobin,[39,40] α_1-acid glycoprotein,[41] and α_1-antitrypsin).[42] Although lectins have been used as sugar detection reagents for decades,[17] the use of multiple lectins for the analysis of biologic samples was not common because of the amount of material and time required for each assay.

Technologic Overview

The lectin microarray made it practically feasible to obtain glycan measurements on a given sample from multiple, different lectins. By incubating samples on an array of lectins and determining the amount of binding to each lectin, a broad profile of the glycans present in the sample can be rapidly obtained with minimal sample consumption. This approach has many advantages over standard methods of glycan analysis, such as reduced cost, time, and sample consumption, with increased reproducibility. An additional advantage is that lectins can provide information about linkages between monosaccharides (eg, whether the alpha or beta configuration), which is not discernable using mass spectrometry analysis.

Some challenges accompany the use of lectin microarrays. One is the question of specificity. Lectins cannot give exact structural information, but rather mainly provide information about terminal structures. Moreover, the specificities of some lectins are incompletely understood and may involve more than one particular structure. Some have suggested that through the use of many lectins, the analysis of an overall lectin-binding profile can overcome some of the ambiguities associated with lectin binding,[43] although the effectiveness of such a strategy has not been demonstrated. Another challenge can be detection sensitivity, because lectin-glycan interactions are weak compared with DNA-RNA or antibody-antigen hybrids. Standard washing protocols developed for protein or DNA microarrays may result in the significant loss of binding. An evanescent-field fluorescence strategy is a promising solution,[44] because it allows the sensitive, real-time observation of monovalent lectin-oligosaccharide interactions under equilibrium conditions without the requirement of washing. The optimization of this method enabled the detection of glycoproteins down to a 100 pm concentration.[45]

The initial demonstrations of lectin microarrays[46,47] used standard arraying methods that had been developed for DNA and protein microarrays. Lectins were printed on aldehyde- or epoxide-derivatized glass slides to achieve covalent immobilization, or were linked by biotin-streptavidin bridges on photoactivatable dextran-coated slides. Another lectin array used the noncovalent suspension of lectins in an aqueous hydrogel matrix,[48] which may better preserve the conformation and activity of lectins relative to binding on planar surfaces. The arrayed lectins were hybridized with samples (eg, glycoproteins) that were directly labeled with a fluorescent tag or that were recognized by a labeled detection reagent.

Studies of Protein Glycosylation

The major application of lectin microarrays has been to investigate rapidly the glycosylation of purified glycoproteins, which were incubated on the arrays. For example, Kuno and coworkers[44] used arrays containing 39 lectins to detect glycosylation differences between various glycoproteins and changes in glycosylation induced by treatment with glycosidases. The incubation of purified proteins, as opposed to mixtures of proteins, is important to simplify the interpretation of the data, so that one may know the identity of the protein binding each lectin. Others have demonstrated the incubation of complex mixtures of proteins onto lectin arrays, however, achieving a summary view of a cell "glycome." Pilobello and coworkers[49] used a ratiometric approach to examining changes in bacterial cell-surface glycomes. Isolated membrane proteins from two bacterial cultures were differentially labeled with Cy3 and Cy5 fluorescent dyes and coincubated on arrays containing up to 58 different lectins. The Cy3/Cy5 ratio at each spot provided a sensitive indicator of differences between the cultures and allowed for normalization between arrays. This analysis enabled the observation of glycosylation changes occurring in response to cell differentiation. The evanescent-field fluorescence method mentioned previously also was applicable to the study of crude glycoproteins extracted from mammalian cells.[50] Although the approach of incubating multiple proteins on lectin arrays offers a summary view of the glycan structures on a cell, it has the disadvantage of integrating information from all proteins, so that glycan changes that occur only on a subset of proteins may be lost in a background of nonchanging proteins.

Cell Surface Glycosylation

A potentially simpler and more direct view of cell-surface glycosylation has been achieved by incubating live cells on the surfaces of lectin microarrays. The use of whole cells as opposed to cell extracts has an advantage of preserving higher-order structures, which may be biologically significant and important for lectin binding. Early work by Zheng and colleagues[51] used covalent immobilization of lectins on self-assembled monolayers that were functionalized with NHS. Cultured cells were incubated on the spotted lectins, and the binding of the cells to the lectins was visualized with an inverted microscope. The gold base substrate was thin enough to allow the imaging. The authors showed differences in the glycosylation of the two cell types. In later work by the same group,[52] the authors used this technology to explore glycan differences between normal and breast cancer cell lines. Significant variation in glycosylation was identified that correlated with metastatic potential and metastatic location preference.

Lectin microarrays also were used to examine dynamic changes to E coli bacterial glycosylation.[53] The bacteria were labeled with a dye that binds to DNA to allow detection by fluorescence after incubation on the arrays. The authors could distinguish E coli strains based on glycosylation and could observe growth-dependent variation in glycosylation on particular strains. Lectin arrays using evanescent-field fluorescence, as described earlier,[44] were used to examine dynamic changes to the cell surfaces glycomes of mammalian cells that had been fluorescently labeled with a DNA-binding dye.[54] Alterations in lectin-binding patterns were seen in glycosylation-defective mutants of CHO cells and in splenocytes from mice with a genetic knockout of a glycosyltransferase gene. Changes in cell surface glycosylation associated with erythroblast differentiation also were observed. Another study using arrays of 94 lectins and a similar detection method examined the lectin-binding signatures of 24 different human cell lines and predicted functional phenotypes based on lectin-binding profiles.[55]

ANTIBODY-LECTIN SANDWICH MICROARRAYS

Another array-based glycoproteomics method is the antibody-lectin sandwich microarray. The value of antibody-lectin sandwich microarrays for glycoproteomics studies is that they provide precise measurements of glycan levels on specific proteins captured directly from biologic samples. This capability enables detailed views of how glycans on particular proteins change in association with disease states or sample conditions. Previous methods did not practically allow that type of investigation.

Studies using enzymatic, chromatographic, and mass spectrometry methods have been very effective for providing detailed information about glycan structures in individual samples, but because of high sample consumption, low throughput, or low reproducibility, such studies did not reveal how frequently particular glycans on particular proteins appear, how closely they are associated with particular disease states, or the distribution of protein carriers on which they appear. Affinity-based methods, using reagents, such as lectins or glycan-binding antibodies to detect glycans, can provide that information, because one may reproducibly measure the glycan levels over multiple samples. Although affinity-based glycosylation studies do not provide the structural detail provided by mass spectrometry and enzymatic methods, they can provide information about the biologic variation of a particular motif.

The method starts with an antibody microarray, essentially identical to those developed for multiplexed protein analyses (see **Fig. 1**).[56] The antibodies on the array can be chosen to target various glycoproteins. A complex biologic sample is incubated on the array, resulting in the capture of glycoproteins by the antibodies. The next step is to probe the glycans on the captured proteins using labeled lectins. The amount of lectin binding at each capture antibody indicates the amount of a particular glycan on the proteins captured by each antibody. A variety of lectins could be used on a given sample to probe several different types of glycans. Glycan-binding antibodies also could be used as detection reagents, such as those raised against the Thomsen-Friedenreich antigens[57] or the Lewis blood-group structures.[58] Antibody-lectin sandwich arrays are similar to previous approaches using lectins in the capture or detection of proteins in microtiter plates,[59] but they harness the power of microarrays to provide high-information content in low-sample volumes.

To interpret the amount of glycan on a protein properly, one must also know the underlying protein concentration. That complementary information may be conveniently obtained using antibody microarrays in a standard sandwich assay format to detect core protein levels (**Fig. 2**). A sample may be incubated multiple times on replicate microarrays, each time probed with a different lectin, to characterize glycan levels (see **Fig. 2**B), or with antibodies, to characterize protein levels (see **Fig. 2**A). A previous study[60] showed the value of using both formats to detect glycosylation differences between samples (see **Fig. 2**C).

The ability to probe each sample multiple times, and to probe many samples (as is required for clinical studies), requires the ability to run many samples efficiently and to consume small sample volumes in each assay. A practical method for the high-throughput processing of low-volume microarrays was demonstrated earlier.[61] Multiple, replicate microarrays are printed onto a microscope slide, and the arrays are separated from one another by hydrophobic, wax borders that are precisely imprinted onto the slide. The borders are imprinted using a device (The Gel Company, San Francisco, California) that elevates a stamp out of a wax bath, which sits atop a hotplate to melt the wax, to contact a microscope slide suspended above the wax bath (**Fig. 3**A). The wax borders prevent liquid from spilling from one array to another, and they remain on the slide throughout the processing steps and the fluorescence scanning (**Fig. 3**B). Any size or pattern of arrays could be accommodated by using the appropriate stamp (**Fig. 3**C). A high-throughput strategy using this format is to incubate sets of samples in a randomized order on a microscope slide and then probe the captured proteins on the slide with a lectin (**Fig. 3**D). Such a strategy has been used for high-throughput antibody array processing in multiple studies.[60,62,63]

Ongoing studies are applying this technology in various ways. One application is the profiling of glycan changes on particular proteins in various disease states, to identify those most associated with disease and to develop new biomarkers. Unpublished

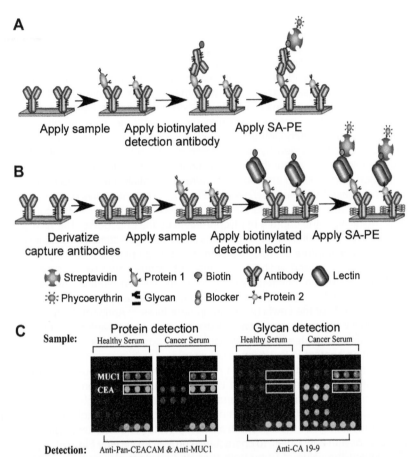

Fig. 2. Complementary detection of protein levels and glycan levels on captured proteins using antibody arrays. (*A*) Array-based sandwich assays for protein detection. Multiple antibodies are immobilized on a planar support, and the captured proteins are probed using biotinylated detection antibodies, followed by fluorescence detection using phycoerythrin-labeled streptavidin. (*B*) Glycan detection on antibody arrays. This format is similar to the previous one, but the detection reagents target the glycans on the captured proteins rather than the core proteins. The glycans on the immobilized antibodies are chemically derivatized to prevent lectin binding to those glycans. (*C*) Detection of differential glycosylation. A healthy patient serum sample and a cancer patient serum sample were incubated on each pair of arrays (same two samples in each pair). The boxes indicate the capture antibodies targeting MUC1 and CEA. The arrays were detected using either a mixture of two antibodies to detect the MUC1 and CEA core proteins (*left array in each pair*) or an antibody detecting the CA 19-9 carbohydrate epitope (*right array in each pair*). The data show equivalent core protein levels between the healthy and cancer serum, but high levels of the CA 19-9 glycan in the cancer serum. The other spots showing signal are control proteins or other proteins containing the CA 19-9 epitope.

data in the authors' laboratory show that certain glycans on particular serum proteins are altered in pancreatic cancer more frequently than the underlying core protein. Because of that relationship, the measurement of the glycan on the protein performs better as a biomarker than the measurement of the protein. The same study also

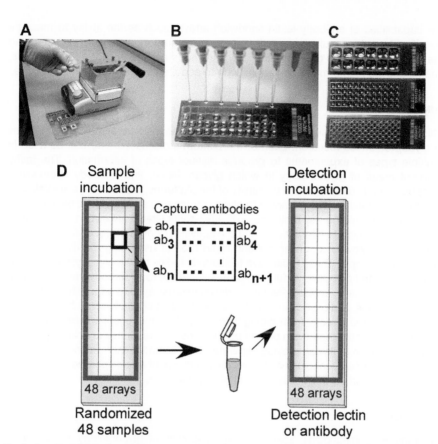

Fig. 3. Practical, high-throughput processing of antibody microarrays. (*A*) Imprinting hydrophobic boundaries. Wax is melted by the hotplate under the bath, and a slide is inserted upside-down into the holder. Bringing the lever forward raises a stamp out of the wax bath to touch the slide, imprinting the design onto the slide to form borders around multiple arrays. Two stamps are shown in front of the machine. (*B*) Loading samples onto a slide containing 48 arrays. The arrays are spaced by 4.5 mm, which is compatible with the 9-mm spacing of standard multichannel pipettes. (*C*) Samples loaded onto slides containing 12 (top), 48 (middle), and 192 (bottom) arrays (96 samples loaded). (*D*) Strategy for profiling glycans in multiple samples. A total of 48 or 60 identical microarrays are printed on one microscope slide, segregated by hydrophobic boundaries. A set of serum samples is incubated on the arrays in a random order, and each slide is probed with a single antibody or lectin.

provides information on the prevalence of glycan alterations in various patient populations, which was not known before because of the aforementioned limitations of conventional glycobiology methods. Another application of this technology is the study of glycan changes induced by various perturbations to cultured cells. For example, the authors have examined the effects of proinflammatory stimuli on the glycan structures of mucins secreted by cancer cells. They found that the induced glycan structures are similar to those observed in clinical samples from pancreatic cancer patients, suggesting that cancer-associated glycans can arise in response to a proinflammatory tumor microenvironment. These types of studies show how the capabilities of antibody-lectin sandwich arrays, such as the ability to measure specific glycans on multiple, specific proteins captured from biologic samples, and the ability to measure changes precisely between samples in those glycan levels, enable access to information that is difficult to acquire using conventional methods.

SUMMARY

This article provides insights into how microarray platforms are stimulating advances in glycoproteomics research. Each of the platforms discussed here can be used in multiple types of experiments to produce distinct types of information. The many different areas of glycobiology in which glycan, lectin, and antibody microarrays have been applied testify to the versatility of the platforms. Glycan arrays are valuable for studying protein and cell binding to glycan structures, and they have been used to study glycan-binding specificities, disease-associated antiglycan antibodies, microbe-carbohydrate interactions, and the activities of glycan-processing enzymes. Lectin arrays provide a convenient and rapid tool for assessing the overall glycan content of a sample. These tools have facilitated studies on the glycosylation of purified proteins and complex mixtures of proteins and the total carbohydrate content of cell surfaces. Finally, antibody-lectin sandwich microarrays are an additional tool for glycoproteomics, and provide information about the carbohydrate on multiple, distinct proteins captured directly from biologic samples. This tool enables views of glycan variation on specific proteins in patient populations or in response to changing conditions. All of these tools can provide experimental information that was not obtainable using conventional technologies. The increased usage of these approaches is anticipated to drive further major advances in glycoproteomics.

REFERENCES

1. Varki A, Cummings R, Esko J, et al. Essentials of glycobiology. Cold Spring Harbor (NY): Cold Spring Harbor Laboratory Press; 1999.
2. Dube DH, Bertozzi CR. Glycans in cancer and inflammation: potential for therapeutics and diagnostics. Nat Rev Drug Discov 2005;4(6):477–88.
3. Dennis JW, Granovsky M, Warren CE. Glycoprotein glycosylation and cancer progression. Biochim Biophys Acta 1999;1473(1):21–34.
4. Fuster MM, Esko JD. The sweet and sour of cancer: glycans as novel therapeutic targets. Nat Rev Cancer 2005;5(7):526–42.
5. Schena M, Shalon D, Davis RW, et al. Quantitative monitoring of gene expression patterns with a complementary DNA microarray. Science 1995;270(5235): 467–70.
6. Hirabayashi J, Hashidate T, Arata Y, et al. Oligosaccharide specificity of galectins: a search by frontal affinity chromatography. Biochim Biophys Acta 2002; 1572(2–3):232–54.
7. Culf AS, Cuperlovic-Culf M, Ouellette RJ. Carbohydrate microarrays: survey of fabrication techniques. OMICS 2006;10(3):289–310.
8. Wang D. Carbohydrate microarrays. Proteomics 2003;3(11):2167–75.
9. Houseman BT, Mrksich M. Carbohydrate arrays for the evaluation of protein binding and enzymatic modification. Chem Biol 2002;9(4):443–54.
10. Park S, Shin I. Fabrication of carbohydrate chips for studying protein-carbohydrate interactions. Angew Chem Int Ed Engl 2002;41(17):3180–2.
11. Fazio F, Bryan MC, Blixt O, et al. Synthesis of sugar arrays in microtiter plate. J Am Chem Soc 2002;124(48):14397–402.

12. Wang D, Liu S, Trummer BJ, et al. Carbohydrate microarrays for the recognition of cross-reactive molecular markers of microbes and host cells. Nat Biotechnol 2002;20(3):275–81.

13. Fukui S, Feizi T, Galustian C, et al. Oligosaccharide microarrays for high-throughput detection and specificity assignments of carbohydrate-protein interactions. Nat Biotechnol 2002;20(10):1011–7.

14. Willats WG, Rasmussen SE, Kristensen T, et al. Sugar-coated microarrays: a novel slide surface for the high-throughput analysis of glycans. Proteomics 2002;2(12):1666–71.

15. Xia B, Kawar ZS, Ju T, et al. Versatile fluorescent derivatization of glycans for glycomic analysis. Nat Methods 2005;2(11):845–50.

16. Blixt O, Head S, Mondala T, et al. Printed covalent glycan array for ligand profiling of diverse glycan binding proteins. Proc Natl Acad Sci U S A 2004;101(49):17033–8.

17. Rudiger H, Gabius HJ. Plant lectins: occurrence, biochemistry, functions and applications. Glycoconj J 2001;18(8):589–613.

18. Manimala JC, Roach TA, Li Z, et al. High-throughput carbohydrate microarray analysis of 24 lectins. Angew Chem Int Ed Engl 2006;45(22):3607–10.

19. Manimala JC, Roach TA, Li Z, et al. High-throughput carbohydrate microarray profiling of 27 antibodies demonstrates widespread specificity problems. Glycobiology 2007;17(8):17C–23C.

20. Manimala JC, Li Z, Jain A, et al. Carbohydrate array analysis of anti-Tn antibodies and lectins reveals unexpected specificities: implications for diagnostic and vaccine development. Chembiochem 2005;6(12):2229–41.

21. Moller I, Marcus SE, Haeger A, et al. High-throughput screening of monoclonal antibodies against plant cell wall glycans by hierarchical clustering of their carbohydrate microarray binding profiles. Glycoconj J 2008;25(1):37–48.

22. Huang CY, Thayer DA, Chang AY, et al. Carbohydrate microarray for profiling the antibodies interacting with Globo H tumor antigen. Proc Natl Acad Sci U S A 2006;103(1):15–20.

23. Lawrie CH, Marafioti T, Hatton CS, et al. Cancer-associated carbohydrate identification in Hodgkin's lymphoma by carbohydrate array profiling. Int J Cancer 2006;118(12):3161–6.

24. Wang CC, Huang YL, Ren CT, et al. Glycan microarray of Globo H and related structures for quantitative analysis of breast cancer. Proc Natl Acad Sci U S A 2008;105(33):11661–6.

25. Wang D, Carroll GT, Turro NJ, et al. Photogenerated glycan arrays identify immunogenic sugar moieties of *Bacillus anthracis* exosporium. Proteomics 2007;7(2):180–4.

26. Blixt O, Hoffmann J, Svenson S, et al. Pathogen specific carbohydrate antigen microarrays: a chip for detection of *Salmonella* O-antigen specific antibodies. Glycoconj J 2008;25(1):27–36.

27. Stevens J, Blixt O, Glaser L, et al. Glycan microarray analysis of the hemagglutinins from modern and pandemic influenza viruses reveals different receptor specificities. J Mol Biol 2006;355(5):1143–55.

28. Disney MD, Seeberger PH. The use of carbohydrate microarrays to study carbohydrate-cell interactions and to detect pathogens. Chem Biol 2004;11(12):1701–7.

29. Park S, Lee MR, Pyo SJ, et al. Carbohydrate chips for studying high-throughput carbohydrate-protein interactions. J Am Chem Soc 2004;126(15):4812–9.

30. Park S, Shin I. Carbohydrate microarrays for assaying galactosyltransferase activity. Org Lett 2007;9(9):1675–8.
31. Blixt O, Allin K, Bohorov O, et al. Glycan microarrays for screening sialyltransferase specificities. Glycoconj J 2008;25(1):59–68.
32. Sharon N, Lis H. History of lectins: from hemagglutinins to biological recognition molecules. Glycobiology 2004;14(11):53R–62R.
33. Sharon N, Lis H. Lectins as cell recognition molecules. Science 1989;246(4927): 227–34.
34. Sharon N, Lis H. The structural basis for carbohydrate recognition by lectins. Adv Exp Med Biol 2001;491:1–16.
35. Sharon N. Lectins: carbohydrate-specific reagents and biological recognition molecules. J Biol Chem 2007;282(5):2753–64.
36. Osako M, Yonezawa S, Siddiki B, et al. Immunohistochemical study of mucin carbohydrates and core proteins in human pancreatic tumors. Cancer 1993; 71(7):2191–9.
37. Satomura Y, Sawabu N, Takemori Y, et al. Expression of various sialylated carbohydrate antigens in malignant and nonmalignant pancreatic tissues. Pancreas 1991;6(4):448–58.
38. Shimizu K, Katoh H, Yamashita F, et al. Comparison of carbohydrate structures of serum alpha-fetoprotein by sequential glycosidase digestion and lectin affinity electrophoresis. Clin Chim Acta 1996;254(1):23–40.
39. Thompson S, Cantwell BM, Cornell C, et al. Abnormally-fucosylated haptoglobin: a cancer marker for tumour burden but not gross liver metastasis. Br J Cancer 1991;64(2):386–90.
40. Okuyama N, Ide Y, Nakano M, et al. Fucosylated haptoglobin is a novel marker for pancreatic cancer: a detailed analysis of the oligosaccharide structure and a possible mechanism for fucosylation. Int J Cancer 2006;118:2803–8.
41. van Dijk W, Havenaar EC, Brinkman-van der Linden EC. Alpha 1-acid glycoprotein (orosomucoid): pathophysiological changes in glycosylation in relation to its function. Glycoconj J 1995;12(3):227–33.
42. Thompson S, Guthrie D, Turner GA. Fucosylated forms of alpha-1-antitrypsin that predict unresponsiveness to chemotherapy in ovarian cancer. Br J Cancer 1988; 58(5):589–93.
43. Hirabayashi J. Lectin-based structural glycomics: glycoproteomics and glycan profiling. Glycoconj J 2004;21(1–2):35–40.
44. Kuno A, Uchiyama N, Koseki-Kuno S, et al. Evanescent-field fluorescence-assisted lectin microarray: a new strategy for glycan profiling. Nat Methods 2005; 2(11):851–6.
45. Uchiyama N, Kuno A, Tateno H, et al. Optimization of evanescent-field fluorescence-assisted lectin microarray for high-sensitivity detection of monovalent oligosaccharides and glycoproteins. Proteomics 2008;8(15):3042–50.
46. Pilobello KT, Krishnamoorthy L, Slawek D, et al. Development of a lectin microarray for the rapid analysis of protein glycopatterns. Chembiochem 2005;6(6): 985–9.
47. Angeloni S, Ridet JL, Kusy N, et al. Glycoprofiling with micro-arrays of glycoconjugates and lectins. Glycobiology 2005;15(1):31–41.
48. Koshi Y, Nakata E, Yamane H, et al. A fluorescent lectin array using supramolecular hydrogel for simple detection and pattern profiling for various glycoconjugates. J Am Chem Soc 2006;128(32):10413–22.

49. Pilobello KT, Slawek DE, Mahal LK. A ratiometric lectin microarray approach to analysis of the dynamic mammalian glycome. Proc Natl Acad Sci U S A 2007; 104(28):11534–9.
50. Ebe Y, Kuno A, Uchiyama N, et al. Application of lectin microarray to crude samples: differential glycan profiling of lec mutants. J Biochem 2006;139(3): 323–7.
51. Zheng T, Peelen D, Smith LM. Lectin arrays for profiling cell surface carbohydrate expression. J Am Chem Soc 2005;127(28):9982–3.
52. Chen S, Zheng T, Shortreed MR, et al. Analysis of cell surface carbohydrate expression patterns in normal and tumorigenic human breast cell lines using lectin arrays. Anal Chem 2007;79(15):5698–702.
53. Hsu KL, Pilobello KT, Mahal LK. Analyzing the dynamic bacterial glycome with a lectin microarray approach. Nat Chem Biol 2006;2(3):153–7.
54. Tateno H, Uchiyama N, Kuno A, et al. A novel strategy for mammalian cell surface glycome profiling using lectin microarray. Glycobiology 2007;17(10):1138–46.
55. Tao SC, Li Y, Zhou J, et al. Lectin microarrays identify cell-specific and functionally significant cell surface glycan markers. Glycobiology 2008;18(10):761–9.
56. Haab BB, Dunham MJ, Brown PO. Protein microarrays for highly parallel detection and quantitation of specific proteins and antibodies in complex solutions. Genome Biol 2001;2(2):RESEARCH0004.
57. Kjeldsen T, Clausen H, Hirohashi S, et al. Preparation and characterization of monoclonal antibodies directed to the tumor-associated O-linked sialosyl-2—6 alpha-N-acetylgalactosaminyl (sialosyl-Tn) epitope. Cancer Res 1988;48(8): 2214–20.
58. Hanisch FG, Hanski C, Hasegawa A. Sialyl Lewis(x) antigen as defined by monoclonal antibody AM-3 is a marker of dysplasia in the colonic adenoma-carcinoma sequence. Cancer Res 1992;52(11):3138–44.
59. Thompson S, Stappenbeck R, Turner GA. A multiwell lectin-binding assay using lotus tetragonolobus for measuring different glycosylated forms of haptoglobin. Clin Chim Acta 1989;180(3):277–84.
60. Chen S, LaRoche T, Hamelinck D, et al. Multiplexed analysis of glycan variation on native proteins captured by antibody microarrays. Nat Methods 2007;4(5): 437–44.
61. Forrester S, Kuick R, Hung KE, et al. Low-volume, high-throughput sandwich immunoassays for profiling plasma proteins in mice: identification of early-stage systemic inflammation in a mouse model of intestinal cancer. Mol Oncol 2007;1: 216–25.
62. Orchekowski R, Hamelinck D, Li L, et al. Antibody microarray profiling reveals individual and combined serum proteins associated with pancreatic cancer. Cancer Res 2005;65(23):11193–202.
63. Gao WM, Kuick R, Orchekowski RP, et al. Distinctive serum protein profiles involving abundant proteins in lung cancer patients based upon antibody microarray analysis. BMC Cancer 2005;5:110–20.
64. Patwa TH, Zhao J, Anderson MA, et al. Screening of glycosylation patterns in serum using natural glycoprotein microarrays and multi-lectin fluorescence detection. Anal Chem 2006;78(18):6411–21.
65. Zhao J, Patwa TH, Qiu W, et al. Glycoprotein microarrays with multi-lectin detection: unique lectin binding patterns as a tool for classifying normal, chronic pancreatitis and pancreatic cancer sera. J Proteome Res 2007;6(5):1864–74.

Autoantibody Profiling for Cancer Detection

Ji Qiu, PhD, Sam Hanash, MD, PhD*

KEYWORDS

• Antibody • Tumor antigen • Cancer detection • Proteomics
• Protein microarray

It is widely appreciated that making major inroads in the fight against cancer is going to depend, in part, on early detection. Detecting cancers based on serum profiling is a particularly attractive concept because a single draw of blood would allow screening for different cancers. There is increasing evidence for a humoral immune response to cancer in humans, as demonstrated by the identification of antibodies against a number of tumor antigens in patients with various tumor types.[1–7] Proteins not present in normal cells may elicit a host immune response that affords a dramatic amplification of signal in the form of antibodies relative to the amount of the corresponding antigen. The immune response occurs early during tumor development and as a result the presence of autoantibodies against tumor antigens in serum might provide an effective means for cancer screening and early diagnosis.

One of the most investigated humoral immune response targets in cancer is the tumor suppressor p53. The p53 gene plays a critical role in maintaining genomic integrity and the p53 pathway is frequently inactivated in almost all common cancer types.[8–10] In 1982, Crawford and colleagues[11] first demonstrated the presence of antibodies against human p53 proteins in 9% of breast patient sera. Subsequently, anti-p53 autoantibodies were detected in patients with a variety of cancers including ovarian, liver, colon, lung, pancreas, and prostate.[12–14] Poor prognosis was shown to be associated with the occurrence of antibodies against p53 among colon cancer patients.[15] Although there is a strong correlation between p53 missense mutations and p53 autoantibodies, some patients have antibodies in the absence of detectable p53 mutations, suggesting that overexpression of wild-type p53 may be sufficient to induce a humoral response. The prevalence of anti-p53 antibodies ranges from 3% to 30% depending on the cancer type. Although it is unlikely that cancer or precancerous conditions can be screened for or diagnosed based only on the detection of p53 antibodies, it is likely that the identification of panels of antigens that induce a humoral response in a cancer type will allow detection of cancer at an early stage.

Division of Public Health Sciences, Fred Hutchinson Cancer Research Center, 1100 Fairview N, M5-C800, Seattle, WA 98109, USA
* Corresponding author.
E-mail address: shanash@fhcrc.org (S. Hanash).

Clin Lab Med 29 (2009) 31–46
doi:10.1016/j.cll.2009.01.002
0272-2712/09/$ – see front matter © 2009 Elsevier Inc. All rights reserved.

CLASSIFICATION OF TUMOR ANTIGENS

Tumor antigens can be loosely categorized into four groups: (1) tumor antigens encoded by genes that are linked to tumorigenesis (eg, L-*myc*, c-*myb*, p21 *ras*, HER2/neu, cyclin B1, survivin, livin);[16–22] (2) tumor antigens encoded by genes referred to as "cancer/testis antigens" whose expression is restricted to tumors and germ cells;[23] (3) tumor antigens encoded by genes that are mutated in tumors (eg, p53);[24,25] and (4) tumor antigens encoded by genes whose protein products exhibit aberrant post-translational modifications, such as glycosylation or proteolytic cleavage (eg, annexin I, calreticulin).[26,27]

It is not clear why certain proteins can elicit an autoantibody response with tumor development. The mechanisms responsible for induction of immune reactivity against tumor antigens are ill defined.[28] The diversity of tumor antigens may indicate different underlying mechanisms for the autoantibody response directed against them. Although tumor antigens expressed on the cell surface are readily accessible for an immune response, intracellular tumor antigens may become immunogenic as a result of distinct processes associated with tumor development and progression including apoptosis and inflammation, which affect antigen presentation and promote a humoral immune response.

For most antigens identified to date, only a subset of patients with a tumor type develops a humoral response to a particular antigen. Tumors exhibit substantial heterogeneity in protein expression, which may partially explain why heterogeneity in the immune response to particular antigens may occur. Other factors, such as major histocompatibility complex (MHC) polymorphisms, may also influence the immune response against a particular antigen.

STRATEGIES FOR IDENTIFICATION OF TUMOR ANTIGENS

Ever since the early observations of cancer immunity, efforts have been made to identify antigens that can trigger a humoral immune response. Early attempts[29–32] relied on an approach referred to as "autologous typing" with a focus on cell-surface antigens, whereby cancer patient sera were reacted with autologous cancer cells. Although several antigens profiled by this approach were defined later,[33,34] it was difficult to purify these antigens for further characterization partially because of the low titers of cancer autoantibodies. Advances in biochemical and molecular biologic techniques have been applied to the discovery of novel tumor antigens resulting in substantial expansion of the tumor antigen repertoire. The potential clinical use of individual antigens has been limited, however, because of poor predictive value. There is a substantial need to develop novel technologies to discover tumor antigen marker panels with the specificity and sensitivity necessary for early screening and diagnosis of cancer. A brief discussion on current strategies for the detection of tumor antigens that induce a humoral immune response follows.

A Candidate-Based Approach

A targeted strategy with predefined candidates is a trial and error approach. A candidate antigen can be "guessed" and "tested" by ELISA or Western blot analysis. For example, because cytoplasmic tyrosine kinase (cSrc) was found to be overexpressed, activated, and in some cases mutated in carcinoma, it was investigated as a tumor antigen. Autoantibodies against three proteins (cSrc; Fyn, another member of the Src family not found to be activated in cancer; and Csk, a COOH-terminal Src tyrosine kinase that downregulates cSrc activity) were assessed by ELISA. Although no autoantibodies were detected against cSrc or Fyn, up to 20% of cancer patients with carcinoma had high-affinity autoantibodies against Csk.[35] A requirement for this approach is the availability of antigens, which can be either purified from cancer cell cultures or produced from a recombinant expression source, such as bacteria, yeast, or insect cells. The purity of recombinant proteins could affect assay results.[36]

Affinity-Based Enrichment

A variation on absorption-based assays as an example of affinity-based approaches is a column-based strategy in which two separate affinity columns are prepared from immobilized immunoglobulins (IgG in most cases) isolated from pooled sera from cancer patients or healthy controls. Proteins from cancer cell lysates are first passed through the affinity column coupled with IgG from healthy controls, then through the column coupled with IgG from cancer patients. Proteins bound to the second column are eluted, characterized, and served as candidate tumor antigens for further validation.[37]

Major Histocompatibility Complex II Bound Peptides

The presentation of peptides derived from tumor antigens by MHC class II molecules is a necessary step in the process of humoral immune response. Tumor antigens can be deduced from the sequence of peptides bound to MHC class II molecules. In one study, peptides eluted from HLA-DR molecules on human monocyte-derived dendritic cells that were pulsed with necrotic melanoma cells were sequenced by a combination of two-dimensional capillary liquid chromatography and electrospray ionization tandem mass spectrometry. Peptides originating from potential tumor antigens were identified using this approach including one epitope derived from the melanoma-associated protein melanotransferrin.[38]

Recombinant Escherichia coli/Phage/Combinatorial Libraries

SEREX based on expression library screening has proved to be a useful strategy for tumor antigen identification and has been relied on for studies of many different cancer types.[39] A vast number of entries have been deposited into the Cancer Immunome Database (https://www2.licr.org/CancerImmunomeDB/), which was developed to share tumor antigens discovered using SEREX. In this approach, cancer patient and healthy control sera are used to probe cDNA expression libraries constructed from tumor tissues, cancer cell lines, or testes. Clones that exhibit differential reactivity between the two sera groups[40–43] are isolated and identified. A high-throughput approach has been developed using phage display of cDNA libraries from cancer sources. In one study, a T7 phage display cDNA library was constructed from an ovarian cancer cell line.[44] Four rounds of differential biopanning were performed with negative and positive selection using pooled sera from healthy women and a late-stage ovarian cancer patient. Individual plaques from the selected phage library were arrayed on nitrocellulose membranes and screened with cancer and normal control sera for differential reactivity. A variation on the cDNA library approach is to use random peptide library phage display to select peptides recognized by circulating antibodies in cancer patient sera. This strategy was applied to prostate cancer and resulted in the identification of a member of the heat shock protein family, GRP78, as a tumor antigen.[4]

Proteomic Approaches

Proteomic approaches for tumor antigen identification have been increasingly recognized for canvassing individual proteins in the whole proteome, in their modification states as they occur in cells, for their antigenicity in a high-throughput multiplexed manner. Given that proteins are subject to post-translational modifications, proteomic approaches hold the promise to discover antigens with epitopes that result from post-translational modifications.

The authors initially implemented a proteomic approach for the identification of tumor antigens that elicit a humoral response using two-dimensional polyacrylamide gel electrophoresis (PAGE) to separate cellular proteins from tumor tissue or tumor cell lines and then screening sera from cancer patients for antibodies that react against the separated proteins by Western blotting. Proteins that specifically react with sera from patients with the same tumor type are identified by mass spectrometry. This strategy has been applied to several tumor types leading to the identification of multiple antigens that have potential as cancer markers for early diagnosis through their detection in serum or through serum profiling for corresponding autoantibodies. Some of the identified antigens have moved to an independent validation phase.[7,27,45–48]

In one study, proteins from a pancreatic tumor cell line (Panc-1) were separated by two-dimensional PAGE and transferred onto polyvinylidene fluoride (PVDF) membranes.[48] Sera obtained from 36 newly diagnosed patients with pancreatic cancer, 18 patients with chronic pancreatitis, 33 patients with other types of cancers, and 15 healthy donors were screened individually for the presence of antibodies to Panc-1 pancreatic tumor cell line proteins. Autoantibodies were detected against either one or two calreticulin isoforms identified by mass spectrometry in sera from 21 of 36 patients with pancreatic cancer. One of 18 chronic pancreatitis patients and 1 of 15 healthy controls demonstrated autoantibodies to calreticulin isoform 1; none demonstrated autoantibodies to isoform 2. None of the sera from patients with colon cancer exhibited reactivity against either of the two isoforms. One of 14 sera from lung adenocarcinoma patients demonstrated autoantibodies to calreticulin isoform 1;2 of 14 demonstrated autoantibodies to isoform 2. Calreticulin antibodies were also identified in sera from patients with liver cancer.[26] Remarkably, the isoform that elicits antibodies in liver cancer is different from the isoforms that elicit antibodies detectable in sera from subjects with pancreatic cancer, providing a clear illustration of the merits of a proteomic approach for identification of diagnostic cancer antigens based on the analysis of natural proteins, as opposed to synthetic peptides or re-combinant proteins that do not have representation of the various isoforms present in tumor cells that result from post-translational modifications and processing of proteins.

The major bottleneck for two-dimensional Western blotting has been the laborious nature of preparing two-dimensional gels from lysates followed by transfer of proteins onto membranes for screening with individual sera. This has limited both the number of sera that could be screened and the number of cell lines and tumors for which this screening approach could be applied. The authors have explored a complementary approach for comprehensive analysis of proteins in their modified forms, which is to array protein fractions following liquid-based separation of lysates isolated from tumor cells and tissues for high throughput screening for tumor antigens that react with anti-bodies in patient sera. This type of array is referred to as "natural protein microarray." Proteins in reactive fractions are identified by mass spectrometry.

Although the concept of a "multianalyte microspot immunoassay" system was first proposed back in the late 1980s,[49] it was not until the development and success of DNA microarrays that protein microarrays gained attention, with substantial progress in recent years. Protein microarrays have emerged as a promising approach to meet the pressing need for systematic analysis of thousands of proteins in parallel. Protein microarrays that contain natural proteins derived from tumor cells have the potential to substantially accelerate the pace of discovery of tumor antigens to yield a molecular signature for immune responses directed against protein targets in different types of cancer. In a study of colon cancer, microarrays printed with 1760 distinct protein fractions, prepared from the LoVo colon adenocarcinoma cell line, were hybridized with individual sera.[50] A fraction that exhibited IgG-based reactivity with 9 of 15 colon cancer sera was found to contain ubiquitin C-terminal hydrolase L3 by tandem mass spectrometry (ESI-Q-TOF). The highest levels of ubiquitin C-terminal hydrolase L3 mRNA among the 329 tumors of different types analyzed by DNA microarrays were found in colon tumors. Independent validation by Western blotting demonstrated that ubiquitin C-terminal hydrolase L3 antibodies existed in 19 of 43 sera from patients with colon cancer and in 0 of 54 sera from subjects with lung cancer, colon adenoma, or otherwise healthy. These preliminary findings led to the conclusion that a natural protein microarray approach has the necessary sensitivity and throughput for the identification of tumor antigens that have induced an antibody response in patients with specific cancers. By using protein extracts from a cancer cell line or from one or more tumor tissues, limitations of other approaches based on recombinant proteins or peptides that lack epitopes resulting from post-translational modifications are overcome.

The application of protein microarrays also encompasses the use of recombinant proteins and peptides with the advantage of requirements of minimal volumes of serum for clinical samples, in addition to their high throughput.[51–53]

AUTOANTIBODIES IN LUNG CANCER

Lung cancer is the leading cause of cancer deaths among men and women in the United States. Lung cancer caused an estimated 160,390 deaths in 2007, accounting for 28.7% of all cancer deaths. The chance for a successful treatment is much higher when cancer is diagnosed at an early stage. Lung cancer has been associated with a paraneoplastic cerebellar degeneration syndrome with occurrence of antineuronal antibodies, such as anti-Hu, anti-P/Q-type voltage-gated calcium, and anti-N-type voltage-gated calcium.[54–61] In one study, using recombinant recoverin, a neuronal calcium-binding protein, as an antigen, autoantibodies against recoverin (anti-Rc) were detected by Western blotting in sera from 15% of patients with small cell lung cancer and from 20% of patients with non–small cell lung cancer. Only two anti–Rc-positive cases were observed among 86 patients with nonmalignant pulmonary disorders and none among 50 healthy individuals.[62]

Targeted studies resulted in the discovery of several antibodies against oncogenes, tumor suppressor genes, and genes that are important in cancer development. For example, anti-c-Myc and anti-L-Myc antibodies were reported to occur in 13.2% and 10% lung cancer patients compared with 3.3% and 0% in healthy controls, respectively.[22,63] Several studies of p53 in lung cancer have been reported.[12,64] Although the frequencies of serum p53 antibodies were statistically higher in lung cancer patients than in the control subjects in most studies, the association of antibodies with clinical parameters, such as survival, is still not well-defined.

Survivin and livin are members of the inhibitor of apoptosis protein family and are highly expressed in cancer cells, but show little or no expression in normal tissues. Rohayem and colleagues[65] reported that 21.6% of lung cancer patient sera (N = 51) reacted with purified recombinant survivin in an ELISA. The presence of antibodies against p53 was also tested for the same collection of sera, and four sera from lung cancer patients contained anti-p53 antibodies (7.8%). Yagihashi and colleagues[20] examined the prevalence of anti-livin and anti-survivin antibodies in lung cancer patients with ELISA using recombinant proteins. Nineteen (51.3%) of 37 lung cancer patients were positive for anti-livin antibodies. Thirty-one samples from the same lung cancer patients were also assayed for anti-survivin antibodies. Eighteen patients (58.1%) were positive for anti-survivin antibodies and 21 patients (71%) were positive for antibodies to survivin, livin, or both. Intensity of anti-livin antibody responses did not correlate with intensity of anti-survivin responses.

In another targeted study, Chang and colleagues[66] examined whether serum from non–small cell lung cancer patients exhibited immunoreactivity against the antioxidant enzyme peroxiredoxin-I using Western blotting after their discovery of Prx-I overexpression in non–small cell lung cancer tissue. They found that 25 (47%) of 53 non–small cell lung cancer patient sera had autoantibodies against Prx-I, whereas only four (8%) sera from 50 healthy subjects showed reactivity to Prx-I. Prx-I itself was detected in the sera from 18 (34%) of 53 non–small cell lung cancer patients but in only one serum from 50 controls. Moreover, 17% of non–small cell lung cancer sera were positive for both Prx-I antibody and antigen but none of control sera. It is interesting to note that Prx-I was found to be secreted by lung adenocarcinoma cells (A549 cell line) but not by noncancerous lung cells (BEAS 2B) or breast cancer cells (MCF7).

Tan and coworkers[67] examined antibody frequencies for a panel of seven tumor-associated anitgens (TAAs) (c-myc, cyclin B1, IMP1, Koc, p53, p62, and survivin) in 527 cancer patients (64 breast cancers, 45 colorectal cancers, 91 gastric cancers, 65 hepatocellular carcinomas, 56 lung cancers, and 206 prostate cancers) and 346 healthy controls. Recursive partitioning was used to assess whether each subject could be accurately classified based on his or her antibody reactivity profile to the seven TAAs. In the case of lung cancers, the classification tree had a sensitivity of 0.8 at a specificity of 0.90 when normal means $\pm$ 2 SDs were used as standard cutoffs for immunoassay positivity. Antibody to cyclin B1 was the initial discriminating node for lung cancers.[68]

In 1998, Gure and colleagues[3] first applied SEREX to lung cancer. Serologic analysis of a recombinant cDNA expression library constructed from a lung adenocarcinoma with the autologous patient serum led to the isolation of 20 clones representing 12 different genes. Embryonic neural proteins were identified as tumor antigens by screening cDNA libraries derived from small cell lung cancer cell lines using pooled sera of small cell lung cancer patients.[69] Brass and colleagues[70] screened a cDNA library generated from a lung squamous carcinoma with autologous patient serum and 35 clones representing 19 genes were isolated. Diesinger and colleagues[71] generated two cDNA libraries from squamous cell lung carcinoma and isolated 15 immunogenic antigens (including elF-4 G) using autologous sera. In a follow-up study, antibodies against recombinant elF-4 G were detected in five (15%) of 33 heterologous sera from lung squamous carcinoma patients, but not in 17 control sera from individuals without tumors and 17 sera from patients with squamous cell carcinoma of the head and neck.

Zhong and colleagues[72] introduced the application of T7 phage display libraries to the identification of circulation antibodies to non–small cell lung cancer antigens. Sera from healthy individuals were used for negative selection. Forty-five immunoreactive phage clones were identified as having significant sequence identity with cDNA from known or suspected tumor-associated proteins. Antibodies against five phage-expressed proteins (HSP70, HSP90, p130, GAGE, and BMI-1) were measured using ELISA in patient (N = 40) and control sera (N = 49). HSP70 had the best performance with an area under the curve of 0.73. The combined area under the curve was 0.84. Zhong and colleagues[73] later implemented a protein microarray approach to T7 phage display analysis and identified five genes (GAGE7, BAC clone RP11-499F19,

SEC15L2, PMS2L15, and EEF1A) that have a combined diagnostic accuracy of 88.9%.

Proteomic approaches have led to the identification of tumor antigens in lung cancer. In one study, sera obtained at the time of diagnosis from 64 patients with lung cancer were investigated for the presence of IgG antibodies to A549 adenocarcinoma cell line proteins and to autologous tumor tissue proteins that were separated by two-dimensional gel electrophoresis. Serum from nine of 64 patients with lung cancer (**Table 1**), consisting of six patients with adenocarcinoma, two with squamous cell carcinoma, and one with SCLC, exhibited IgG-based reactivity against a group of three proteins with an estimated molecular weight of 25 kd and with a pI between 5 and 5.6 (**Fig. 1**). Reactivity was specific to IgG1 among the IgG subtypes examined (IgG1–4). The identity of this set of proteins was determined by mass spectrometry after trypsin digestion and corresponded to protein gene product 9.5 (PGP 9.5). The lung cancer specificity of PGP 9.5 autoantibodies was determined by screening sera from 99 patients with other types of cancer and 71 sera from noncancer controls (see **Table 1**). Only one serum in the cancer control group, from a patient with hepatocellular carcinoma, exhibited immunoreactivity against PGP 9.5 proteins. The noncancer control group consisted of sera from 61 healthy subjects, including 15 chronic smokers, and from 10 patients with chronic lung disease. Only one serum (from a healthy postpartum, nonsmoker female subject) exhibited immunoreactivity against PGP 9.5 proteins.

Increased levels of PGP 9.5 mRNA and protein have been previously reported in non–small cell lung cancer tissue based on serial analysis of gene expression and immunohistochemistry.[74,75] To determine the cellular distribution of PGP 9.5 and its possible occurrence as a secreted protein, subcellular compartments from the A549 adenocarcinoma cell line were investigated by Western blotting. PGP 9.5 was readily detected in the membrane and the secreted protein fractions. Interestingly, two sera from lung cancer patients that did not contain autoantibodies against PGP 9.5 exhibited circulating PGP 9.5 protein. Circulating PGP 9.5 protein was not detected in

Table 1
Anti–PGP 9.5 autoantibodies in subject sera

	Number of Subjects	PGP 9.5 Auto AB Positive
Lung cancer	**64**	**9**
Adenocarcinoma	40	6
Squamous cell carcinoma	18	2
Small cell carcinoma	4	1
Large cell carcinoma	2	0
Other types of cancer	**99**	**1**
Brain cancer	14	0
Neuroblastoma	23	0
Breast cancer	11	0
Melanoma	7	0
Liver cancer	44	1
Other controls	**71**	**1**
Healthy nonsmokers	46	1
Chronic smokers	15	0
Chronic lung disease	10	0

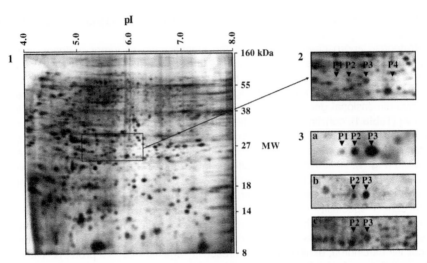

Fig. 1. Two-dimensional PAGE and Western blot analysis of A549 lung adenocarcinoma cell proteins. Panel 1 shows the A549 two-dimensional protein pattern after silver staining. The boxed area is shown on panel 2, in which arrows point to the location of PGP 9.5 forms (spots P1–P3) recognized by sera from patients with lung cancer and the position of the form P4, which is recognized by a polyclonal rabbit anti–PGP 9.5 antiserum that also recognizes P1 to P3. Panel 3 shows close-ups of Western blots from A549 cell proteins (a) and tumor tissue proteins from a patient with lung cancer (b) hybridized with his autologous serum showing reactivity against PGP 9.5 proteins. A close-up of the autologous tumor tissue two-dimensional protein pattern stained with silver nitrate (c) shows P2 and P3 PGP 9.5 variants.

any of the control sera. In all, PGP 9.5 was found to elicit autoantibodies or to occur in circulation among newly diagnosed patients with lung cancer.

In another study following a similar approach as for PGP9.5, a set of sera from 54 newly diagnosed patients with lung cancer and 60 patients with other cancers and from 61 non-cancer controls were investigated. Sera from 60% of patients with lung adenocarcinoma, 33% of patients with squamous cell lung carcinoma, but none of the non-cancer controls had IgG-based reactivity against proteins identified as glycosylated annexins one and II in A549 two-dimensional Western blots (**Table 2**). Positive sera were generally reactive against annexins I and II at the highest serum dilution tested, which was one per 1000. Reactivity was not limited to patients with advanced-stage disease. Sera showed similar reactivity against annexins I and II in autologous tumor protein blots and in blots prepared from normal lung tissue, as in A549-derived blots. Sera from lung cancer patients that exhibited IgG-based reactivity against annexins I or II exhibited reactivity that was specific to IgG1 among the IgG subtypes examined, and also exhibited IgM-based reactivity. None of the sera from other cancer types or from noncancer controls exhibited autoantibodies against annexin II. Sera from six of 60 patients with other types of cancers, namely four of 17 with esophageal cancer, one of 14 with brain tumor, and one of 11 with breast cancer, exhibited annexin reactivity.

Annexin expression in lung tumors was assessed by immunohistochemistry, using monoclonal antiannexin I and II antibodies. Annexin I was abundantly expressed in a diffuse manner in most adenocarcinomas and squamous cell carcinomas. Intense annexin II immunoreactivity was also detected in most tumors in a predominantly

Table 2 Antiannexins I and II autoantibodies in subject sera			
	Number of Subjects	Annexin I Auto Ab Positive	Annexin II Auto Ab Positive
Lung cancer	54	16	18
Adenocarcinoma	30	12	11
Squamous cell carcinoma	18	3	4
Small cell carcinoma	4	1	2
Large cell carcinoma	2	0	1
Other types of cancer	60	6	0
Brain cancer	14	1	0
Breast cancer	11	1	0
Melanoma	7	0	0
Liver cancer	11	0	0
Esophageal cancer	17	4	0
Other controls	61	0	0
Healthy subjects	51	0	0
Chronic lung disease	10	0	0

membranous pattern. There were no appreciable differences in annexin I and II expression, by immunohistochemical analysis, between autoantibody positive and negative lung cancer patients. Interestingly, annexin I was subjected to N- or O-deglycosylation. The resulting products were separated by SDS electrophoresis and analyzed by Western blotting. N-deglycosylation by endoglycosidase F induced a basic shift of the protein, whereas no change was observed after O-glycosidase treatment, compared with untreated annexin I. Two sera were tested that exhibited IgG-based immunoreactivity against annexin I. These sera did not react against endoglycosidase F–treated annexin but exhibited IgG-based immunoreactivity against annexin I after O-glycosidase treatment.

A recent study by Pereira-Faca and colleagues[76] screened two sets of newly diagnosed lung cancer sera for their reactivity by Western blotting with chromatographically fractionated protein extracts from three lung cancer cell lines (A549, H23, and H522). One set consisted of sera from 19 newly diagnosed subjects with lung adenocarcinoma and 19 matched controls. A second independent set consisted of sera from 26 newly diagnosed subjects with lung adenocarcinoma and 24 controls matched for age, gender, and smoking history. One protein that exhibited significant reactivity with both sets of cancer sera ($P = .0008$) was confidently identified by mass spectrometry as 14-3-3 theta. Remarkably, significant autoantibody reactivity against 14-3-3 theta was also observed in an analysis of a third set consisting of 18 prediagnostic lung cancer sera collected as part of the Beta-Carotene and Retinol Efficacy Trial (CARET) cohort study, relative to 19 matched controls ($P = .0042$). A receiver operating characteristic curve constructed with a panel of three proteins consisting of 14-3-3 theta identified in this study, plus annexin 1 and PGP 9.5 proteins previously identified as associated with autoantibodies in lung cancer as described previously, gave a sensitivity of 55% at 95% specificity (area under the curve = 0.838) in discriminating lung cancer at the preclinical stage from matched controls.

Natural protein microarrays[77] were also applied to the discovery of tumor antigens in lung cancer. In one study,[78] the lung adenocarcinoma cell line A549 was relied on to determine reactivity of its arrayed proteins with sera from lung cancer patients and controls. A total of 150 mg of A549 proteins was separated into 20 fractions by isoelectric focusing. Each fraction was subjected to reverse-phase high-performance liquid chromatography and 92 fractions were collected. A total of 1840 fractions were printed in duplicate onto nitrocellulose slides. Slides were hybridized each with a serum sample and autoantibody reactivity was detected by an indirect immunofluorescence method.[79] Two typical images of antigen slides are shown in **Fig. 2**. A distinct reactivity pattern in each slide is clearly observed in a comparison of the two images. A total of 19 lung cancer and 14 control seras were investigated. For each fraction, the number of cancer sera that gave higher fluorescent intensity than the second highest normal serum was determined. The number of fractions expected to have "N" or more patient samples bigger than the second biggest normal was estimated by simulation. **Table 3** provides a summary of the statistical results. The probability that nine or more cancer sera has values for a spot higher than the second largest control is less than 0.008. At this significance level, the number of fractions expected by chance is 15. The number of fractions that fit the criteria was 63, however, which was 4.1 times more than expected by chance alone.

An important promise of autoantibodies to tumor antigens is their potential for early detection. In a recent study, proteins from human lung adenocarcinoma cell line A549 lysates were subjected to extensive fractionation.[80] The resulting 1824 fractions were spotted in duplicate on nitrocellulose-coated slides. The microarrays produced were used in a blinded validation study to determine whether annexin I, PGP 9.5, and 14-3-3 theta antigens previously found to be targets of autoantibodies in newly diagnosed subjects with lung cancer are associated with autoantibodies in sera collected at the presymptomatic stage and to determine whether additional antigens may be identified in prediagnostic sera. Individual sera collected from 85 subjects within a year before a diagnosis of lung cancer and 85 matched controls from the CARET cohort were hybridized to individual microarrays. The evidence obtained indicated the occurrence in lung cancer sera of autoantibodies to annexin I, 14-3-3 theta, and a novel lung cancer antigen, LAMR1, which precede onset of symptoms and diagnosis. The findings do provide supportive evidence for the potential use of autoantibodies for the diagnosis of lung cancer before onset of symptoms.

NORMAL

CANCER

Fig. 2. Two typical slide images. The top one was hybridized with a normal serum sample and the bottom a lung cancer patient serum sample.

Table 3			
Statistical analysis results (M2-statistic)			
	M2-Statistic		
N	**Numbers Obtained Experimentally**	**Numbers Expected by Chance**	**Obtained/Expected**
0	1840	1840	1
1	1655	1474	1.12
2	1262	1050	1.20
3	879	688	1.28
4	607	422	1.44
5	406	244	1.66
6	255	133	1.91
7	174	69	2.53
8	106	34	3.16
9	63	15	4.11
10	34	6	5.21
11	13	3	5.02
12	8	1	8.67
13	4	0	NA
14	0	0	NA
15	0	0	NA
16	0	0	NA
17	0	0	NA

Column 2 shows the number of fractions with "N" or more cancer samples that gave higher intensity than the second largest normal sample obtained from the protein microarray experiment; column 3 shows the number expected by chance; column 4 shows the ratio of the number actually obtained to the number expected by chance. A total of 18 cancer and 15 normal samples were studied.

SUMMARY

The identification of tumor antigens that elicit an antibody-based immune response may be useful in cancer screening and immunotherapy. Clearly, tumors may develop in the presence of this antibody-mediated immune response. It has been increasingly realized that each individual autoantibody marker might have limited use because its classification performance by itself may not meet the requirement of a clinical assay. Identification of panels of tumor antigens that have restricted expression to particular cancer types and that induce autoantibodies, in combination with other clinical modalities, has the potential to yield a molecular signature for blood-based screening and diagnosis. The identification of tumor antigens that have elicited humoral immune responses also has direct relevance to cancer therapeutics because many of these antigens are also involved in cell-mediated immune reactions, which is the principal mechanism for tumor immunity.[81–85]

REFERENCES

1. Stockert E, Jager E, Chen YT, et al. A survey of the humoral immune response of cancer patients to a panel of human tumor antigens. J Exp Med 1998;187: 1349–54.

2. Gourevitch MM, von Mensdorff-Pouilly S, Litvinov SV, et al. Polymorphic epithelial mucin (MUC-1)-containing circulating immune complexes in carcinoma patients. Br J Cancer 1995;72:934–8.
3. Gure AO, Altorki NK, Stockert E, et al. Human lung cancer antigens recognized by autologous antibodies: definition of a novel cDNA derived from the tumor suppressor gene locus on chromosome 3p21.3. Cancer Res 1998;58: 1034–41.
4. Mintz PJ, Kim J, Do K-A, et al. Fingerprinting the circulating repertoire of antibodies from cancer patients. Nat Biotechnol 2003;21:57–63.
5. Hanash S. Harnessing immunity for cancer marker discovery. Nat Biotechnol 2003;21(1):37–8.
6. Dunn GP, Bruce AT, Ikeda H, et al. Cancer immunoediting from immunosurveillance to tumor evasion. Nat Immunol 2002;3:991–8.
7. Prasannan L, Misek DE, Hinderer R, et al. Identification of beta-tubulin isoforms as tumor antigens in neuroblastoma. Clin Cancer Res 2000;6(10):3949–56.
8. Vogelstein B, Lane D, Levine AJ. Surfing the p53 network. Nature 2000; 408(6810):307–10.
9. Harris SL, Levine AJ. The p53 pathway: positive and negative feedback loops. Oncogene 2005;24(17):2899–908.
10. Aylon Y, Oren M. Living with p53, dying of p53. Cell 2007;130(4):597–600.
11. Crawford LV, Pim DC, Bulbrook RD. Detection of antibodies against the cellular protein p53 in sera from patients with breast cancer. Int J Cancer 1982;30(4): 403–8.
12. Soussi T. p53 Antibodies in the sera of patients with various types of cancer: a review. Cancer Res 2000;60(7):1777–88.
13. Angelopoulou K, Diamandis EP, Sutherland DJ, et al. Prevalence of serum antibodies against the p53 tumor suppressor gene protein in various cancers. Int J Cancer 1994;58:480–7.
14. Ohshio G, Suwa H, Imamura M. Clinical implication of anti-p53 antibodies and p53-protein in pancreatic disease. Int J Gastrointest Cancer 2002;31(1–3): 129–35.
15. Houbiers JG, van der Burg SH, van de Watering LM, et al. Antibodies against p53 are associated with poor prognosis of colorectal cancer. Br J Cancer 1995;72(3): 637–41.
16. Ward RL, Hawkins NJ, Coomber D, et al. Antibody immunity to the HER-2/neu oncogenic protein in patients with colorectal cancer. Hum Immunol 1999;60(6): 510–5.
17. Sorokine I, Ben-Mahrez K, Bracone A, et al. Presence of circulating anti-c-myb oncogene product antibodies in human sera. Int J Cancer 1991;47(5):665–9.
18. Cheever MA, Disis ML, Bernhard H, et al. Immunity to oncogenic proteins. Immunol Rev 1995;145:33–59.
19. Covini G, Chan EK, Nishioka M, et al. Immune response to cyclin B1 in hepatocellular carcinoma. Hepatology 1997;25(1):75–80.
20. Yagihashi A, Asanuma K, Kobayashi D, et al. Detection of autoantibodies to livin and survivin in sera from lung cancer patients. Lung Cancer 2005;48(2):217–21.
21. Yagihashi A, Ohmura T, Asanuma K, et al. Detection of autoantibodies to survivin and livin in sera from patients with breast cancer. Clin Chim Acta 2005;362(1–2): 125–30.
22. Yamamoto A, Shimizu E, Ogura T, et al. Detection of auto-antibodies against L-myc oncogene products in sera from lung cancer patients. Int J Cancer 1996;69(4):283–9.

23. Scanlan MJ, Gure AO, Jungbluth AA, et al. Cancer/testis antigens: an expanding family of targets for cancer immunotherapy. Immunol Rev 2002;188(1):22–32.

24. von Brevern MC, Hollstein MC, Cawley HM, et al. Circulating anti-p53 antibodies in esophageal cancer patients are found predominantly in individuals with p53 core domain mutations in their tumors. Cancer Res 1996;56(21):4917–21.

25. Winter SF, Minna JD, Johnson BE, et al. Development of antibodies against p53 in lung cancer patients appears to be dependent on the type of p53 mutation. Cancer Res 1992;52(15):4168–74.

26. Chignard N, Shang S, Wang H, et al. Cleavage of endoplasmic reticulum proteins in hepatocellular carcinoma: detection of generated fragments in patient sera. Gastroenterology 2006;130(7):2010–22.

27. Brichory FM, Misek DE, Yim AM, et al. An immune response manifested by the common occurrence of annexins I and II autoantibodies and high circulating levels of IL-6 in lung cancer. Proc Natl Acad Sci U S A 2001;98(17):9824–9.

28. Zinkernagel RM, Ehl S, Aichele P, et al. Antigen localisation regulates immune responses in a dose- and time-dependent fashion: a geographical view of immune reactivity. Immunol Rev 1997;156:199–209.

29. Old LJ, Chen YT. New paths in human cancer serology. J Exp Med 1998;187(8): 1163–7.

30. Shiku H, Takahashi T, Oettgen HF. Cell surface antigens of human malignant melanoma. II. Serological typing with immune adherence assays and definition of two new surface antigens. J Exp Med 1976;144(4):873–81.

31. Shiku H, Takahashi T, Resnick LA, et al. Cell surface antigens of human malignant melanoma. III. Recognition of autoantibodies with unusual characteristics. J Exp Med 1977;145(3):784–9.

32. Carey TE, Takahashi T, Resnick LA, et al. Cell surface antigens of human malignant melanoma: mixed hemadsorption assays for humoral immunity to cultured autologous melanoma cells. Proc Natl Acad Sci U S A 1976;73(9):3278–82.

33. Real FX, Mattes MJ, Houghton AN, et al. Class 1 (unique) tumor antigens of human melanoma: identification of a 90,000 dalton cell surface glycoprotein by autologous antibody. J Exp Med 1984;160(4):1219–33.

34. Watanabe T, Pukel CS, Takeyama H, et al. Human melanoma antigen AH is an autoantigenic ganglioside related to GD2. J Exp Med 1982;156(6):1884–9.

35. Benistant C, Bourgaux JF, Chapuis H, et al. The COOH-terminal Src kinase Csk is a tumor antigen in human carcinoma. Cancer Res 2001;61(4):1415–20.

36. Schmetzer O, Moldenhauer G, Riesenberg R, et al. Quality of recombinant protein determines the amount of autoreactivity detected against the tumor-associated epithelial cell adhesion molecule antigen: low frequency of antibodies against the natural protein. J Immunol 2005;174(2):942–52.

37. Philip R, Murthy S, Krakover J, et al. Shared immunoproteome for ovarian cancer diagnostics and immunotherapy: potential theranostic approach to cancer. J Proteome Res 2007;6(7):2509–17.

38. Rohn TA, Reitz A, Paschen A, et al. A novel strategy for the discovery of MHC class II-restricted tumor antigens: identification of a melanotransferrin helper T-cell epitope. Cancer Res 2005;65(21):10068–78.

39. Sahin U, Tureci O, Schmitt H, et al. Human neoplasms elicit multiple specific immune responses in the autologous host. Proc Natl Acad Sci U S A 1995; 92(25):11810–3.

40. Preuss KD, Zwick C, Bormann C, et al. Analysis of the B-cell repertoire against antigens expressed by human neoplasms. Immunol Rev 2002; 188(1):43–50.

41. Jager D. Potential target antigens for immunotherapy identified by serological expression cloning (SEREX). Methods Mol Biol 2007;360:319–26.
42. Lee SY, Obata Y, Yoshida M, et al. Immunomic analysis of human sarcoma. Proc Natl Acad Sci U S A 2003;100(5):2651–6.
43. Chen YT, Scanlan MJ, Sahin U, et al. A testicular antigen aberrantly expressed in human cancers detected by autologous antibody screening. Proc Natl Acad Sci U S A 1997;94(5):1914–8.
44. Chatterjee M, Mohapatra S, Ionan A, et al. Diagnostic markers of ovarian cancer by high-throughput antigen cloning and detection on arrays. Cancer Res 2006; 66(2):1181–90.
45. Brichory F, Beer D, Le Naour F, et al. Proteomics-based identification of protein gene product 9.5 as a tumor antigen that induces a humoral immune response in lung cancer. Cancer Res 2001;61(21):7908–12.
46. Le Naour F, Brichory F, Misek DE, et al. A distinct repertoire of autoantibodies in hepatocellular carcinoma identified by proteomic analysis. Mol Cell Proteomics 2002;1(3):197–203.
47. Le Naour F, Misek DE, Krause MC, et al. Proteomics-based identification of RS/DJ-1 as a novel circulating tumor antigen in breast cancer. Clin Cancer Res 2001;7(11):3328–35.
48. Hong SH, Misek DE, Wang H, et al. An autoantibody-mediated immune response to calreticulin isoforms in pancreatic cancer. Cancer Res 2004; 64(15):5504–10.
49. Ekins RP. Multi-analyte immunoassay. J Pharm Biomed Anal 1989;7(2):155–68.
50. Nam MJ, Madoz-Gurpide J, Wang H, et al. Molecular profiling of the immune response in colon cancer using protein microarrays: occurrence of autoantibodies to ubiquitin C-terminal hydrolase L3. Proteomics 2003;3(11):2108–15.
51. Hudson ME, Pozdnyakova I, Haines K, et al. Identification of differentially expressed proteins in ovarian cancer using high-density protein microarrays. Proc Natl Acad Sci U S A 2007;104(44):17494–9.
52. Ramachandran N, Hainsworth E, Bhullar B, et al. Self-assembling protein microarrays. Science 2004;305(5680):86–90.
53. Ramachandran N, Hainsworth E, Demirkan G, et al. On-chip protein synthesis for making microarrays. Methods Mol Biol 2006;328:1–14.
54. Tora M, Graus F, de Bolos C, et al. Cell surface expression of paraneoplastic encephalomyelitis/sensory neuronopathy-associated Hu antigens in small-cell lung cancers and neuroblastomas. Neurology 1997;48(3):735–41.
55. Blaes F, Klotz M, Funke D, et al. Disturbance in the serum IgG subclass distribution in patients with anti-Hu positive paraneoplastic neurological syndromes. Eur J Neurol 2002;9(4):369–72.
56. Monstad SE, Drivsholm L, Storstein A, et al. Hu and voltage-gated calcium channel (VGCC) antibodies related to the prognosis of small-cell lung cancer. J Clin Oncol 2004;22(5):795–800.
57. Wirtz PW, Lang B, Graus F, et al. P/Q-type calcium channel antibodies, Lambert-Eaton myasthenic syndrome and survival in small cell lung cancer. J Neuroimmunol 2005;164(1–2):161–5.
58. Storstein A, Monstad SE, Nakkestad HL, et al. Paraneoplastic antibodies against HuD detected by a sensitive radiobinding assay. J Neurol 2004;251(2):197–203.
59. Altermatt HJ, Rodriguez M, Scheithauer BW, et al. Paraneoplastic anti-Purkinje and type I anti-neuronal nuclear autoantibodies bind selectively to central, peripheral, and autonomic nervous system cells. Lab Invest 1991;65(4): 412–20.

60. Mason WP, Graus F, Lang B, et al. Small-cell lung cancer, paraneoplastic cerebellar degeneration and the Lambert-Eaton myasthenic syndrome. Brain 1997; 120(Pt 8):1279–300.
61. Jankowska R, Witkowska D, Porebska I, et al. Serum antibodies to retinal antigens in lung cancer and sarcoidosis. Pathobiology 2004;71(6):323–8.
62. Bazhin AV, Savchenko MS, Shifrina ON, et al. Recoverin as a paraneoplastic antigen in lung cancer: the occurrence of anti-recoverin autoantibodies in sera and recoverin in tumors. Lung Cancer 2004;44(2):193–8.
63. Yamamoto A, Shimizu E, Takeuchi E, et al. Infrequent presence of anti-c-Myc antibodies and absence of c-Myc oncoprotein in sera from lung cancer patients. Oncology 1999;56(2):129–33.
64. Cioffi M, Vietri MT, Gazzerro P, et al. Serum anti-p53 antibodies in lung cancer: comparison with established tumor markers. Lung Cancer 2001; 33(2–3):163–9.
65. Rohayem J, Diestelkoetter P, Weigle B, et al. Antibody response to the tumor-associated inhibitor of apoptosis protein survivin in cancer patients. Cancer Res 2000;60(7):1815–7.
66. Chang JW, Lee SH, Jeong JY, et al. Peroxiredoxin-I is an autoimmunogenic tumor antigen in non-small cell lung cancer. FEBS Lett 2005;579(13):2873–7.
67. Koziol JA, Zhang JY, Casiano CA, et al. Recursive partitioning as an approach to selection of immune markers for tumor diagnosis. Clin Cancer Res 2003;9: 5120–6.
68. Koziol JA, Zhang JY, Casiano CA, et al. Recursive partitioning as an approach to selection of immune markers for tumor diagnosis. Clin Cancer Res 2003;9(14): 5120–6.
69. Gure AO, Stockert E, Scanlan MJ, et al. Serological identification of embryonic neural proteins as highly immunogenic tumor antigens in small cell lung cancer. Proc Natl Acad Sci U S A 2000;97(8):4198–203.
70. Brass N, Racz A, Bauer C, et al. Role of amplified genes in the production of autoantibodies. Blood 1999;93(7):2158–66.
71. Diesinger I, Bauer C, Brass N, et al. Toward a more complete recognition of immunoreactive antigens in squamous cell lung carcinoma. Int J Cancer 2002; 102(4):372–8.
72. Zhong L, Peng X, Hidalgo GE, et al. Identification of circulating antibodies to tumor-associated proteins for combined use as markers of non-small cell lung cancer. Proteomics 2004;4(4):1216–25.
73. Zhong L, Hidalgo GE, Stromberg AJ, et al. Using protein microarray as a diagnostic assay for non-small cell lung cancer. Am J Respir Crit Care Med 2005; 172(10):1308–14.
74. Hibi K, Liu Q, Beaudry GA, et al. Serial analysis of gene expression in non-small cell lung cancer. Cancer Res 1998;58(24):5690–4.
75. Hibi K, Westra WH, Borges M, et al. PGP9.5 as a candidate tumor marker for non-small-cell lung cancer. Am J Pathol 1999;155(3):711–5.
76. Pereira-Faca SR, Kuick R, Puravs E, et al. Identification of 14-3-3 theta as an antigen that induces a humoral response in lung cancer. Cancer Res 2007;67: 12000–6.
77. Madoz-Gurpide J, Wang H, Misek DE, et al. Protein based microarrays: a tool for probing the proteome of cancer cells and tissues. Proteomics 2001;1(10):1279–87.
78. Qiu J, Madoz-Gurpide J, Misek DE, et al. Development of natural protein microarrays for diagnosing cancer based on an antibody response to tumor antigens. J Proteome Res 2004;3:261–7.

79. Bouwman K, Qiu J, Zhou H, et al. Microarrays of tumor cell derived proteins uncover a distinct pattern of prostate cancer serum immunoreactivity. Proteomics 2003;3(11):2200–7.

80. Qiu J, Choi G, Li L, et al. Occurrence of autoantibodies to annexin I, 14-3-3 Theta and LAMR1 in prediagnostic lung cancer sera. J Clin Oncol 2008;26:5060–6.

81. Jager E, Chen YT, Drijfhout JW, et al. Simultaneous humoral and cellular immune response against cancer-testis antigen NY-ESO-1: definition of human histocompatibility leukocyte antigen (HLA)-A2-binding peptide epitopes. J Exp Med 1998; 187(2):265–70.

82. Nishikawa H, Tanida K, Ikeda H, et al. Role of SEREX-defined immunogenic wild-type cellular molecules in the development of tumor-specific immunity. Proc Natl Acad Sci U S A 2001;98(25):14571–6.

83. Jager D, Jager E, Bert F, et al. Cellular and humoral immune responses of cancer patients to defined tumor antigens. Cancer Chemother Biol Response Modif 2001;19:385–93.

84. Jager D, Karbach J, Pauligk C, et al. Humoral and cellular immune responses against the breast cancer antigen NY-BR-1: definition of two HLA-A2 restricted peptide epitopes. Cancer Immun 2005;5:11.

85. Ayyoub M, Stevanovic S, Sahin U, et al. Proteasome-assisted identification of a SSX-2-derived epitope recognized by tumor-reactive CTL infiltrating metastatic melanoma. J Immunol 2002;168(4):1717–22.

Development and Validation of a Protein-based Signature for the Detection of Ovarian Cancer

Kyongjin Kim, MD, Irene Visintin, BA, Ayesha B. Alvero, MD, Gil Mor, MD, PhD*

KEYWORDS

- Ovarian cancer • Early detection • Leptin • Prolactin
- Osteopontin • Macrophage Inhibitory Factor (MIF)
- Insulin-like Growth Factor-II (IGF-II) multiplex

Epithelial ovarian cancer (EOC) is a complex disease that arises due to genetic alterations related to proliferation, apoptosis, and senescence. The majority of the cases of EOC arise because of sporadic accumulation of genetic damage,[1] but 10% arise in women with a known germ-line mutation in BRCA1 or BRCA2.[2]

The high mortality rate of EOC is because of the lack of a screening strategy for early detection. Such a test would aid in the identification of patients who have early stage disease, which usually presents with vague and nonspecific symptoms. Indeed, 80% of patients are diagnosed with advanced stage disease, and they are usually diagnosed when acute symptoms related to metastasis and bowel obstruction are present.[3,4] A large study in the year 2000 showed that in 1725 women evaluated for EOC, 95% exhibited symptoms only 3 months prior to seeing their physician. The women presented with: abdominal (77%) and gastrointestinal (70%) symptoms, pain (58%), urinary (34%), and pelvic symptoms (26%). Gynecologic symptoms were the least common.[5]

Early detection can significantly improve patient survival. In patients who are diagnosed with early disease (stage I or II), the five-year survival ranges from 60% to 90%, depending on the degree of tumor differentiation.[6,7] However, in patients who have advanced disease, although 80%–90% will initially respond to chemotherapy, less

Financial Disclosure: LabCorp has a license agreement with Yale University for the Multiplex biomarker test. GM is a consultant for Teva pharmaceutical.

Department of Obstetrics, Gynecology and Reproductive Sciences, Reproductive Immunology Unit, Yale University School of Medicine, 333 Cedar Street FMB 301, New Haven, CT 06520, USA
* Corresponding author.
E-mail address: gil.mor@yale.edu (G. Mor).

Clin Lab Med 29 (2009) 47–55
doi:10.1016/j.cll.2009.02.001
0272-2712/09/$ – see front matter © 2009 Elsevier Inc. All rights reserved.

labmed.theclinics.com

than 10%–15% will remain in permanent remission.[8] Although advances in treatment have led to an improved five-year survival rate approaching 45%, overall survival has not been enhanced. Therefore, the discovery of a method for early detection of EOC cancer is crucial.

Although ovarian cancer has a high mortality rate, it is still a relatively uncommon disease. The incidence is no more than 40 per 100,000 per year even in the postmenopausal population.[9] There is therefore a concern that the morbidity (and potentially mortality) associated with complications of surgery for false-positive screening results will outweigh the benefits of early detection in women with true-positive results. To be acceptable for this population, a screening strategy must achieve a minimum positive predictive value (PPV) of 10% (ie, no more than nine false positives for each true positive). To achieve this 10% PPV target when screening the general population of postmenopausal women with an incidence of 40/100,000/year, a screening test for ovarian cancer will need to achieve a minimum of 99.6% specificity.

The lack of specific markers for ovarian cancer makes it difficult to achieve the clinical objective of early detection using noninvasive screening methods. Until now, screening consisted of physical examination, ultrasound, and/or cancer antigen 125 (CA-125). However, when taken together, these parameters only detect 30%–45% of early disease. Thus, the identification of other cancer-specific markers for early detection of EOC is essential to improve our ability to accurately detect premalignant changes or early stage EOC in asymptomatic women.[10]

Because currently available strategies for the prevention of ovarian cancer have not proven as effective as interventions targeted against other cancers in women, there has been tremendous interest in using genomics and proteomics to identify potential new markers that can be used in early detection of this disease.[11] Technological developments have led to rapidly expanding knowledge about gene expression and protein patterns in ovarian cancer. Genomic tests have been used for the presence or quantity of the product of a single gene, tests for inherited or acquired mutations in genes that convey an increased risk of developing ovarian cancer, or that predict differential responses to therapy (polymorphisms of breast cancer genes 1 and 2 (BRCA1/2)), tests for quantitative expression of either single genes or multiple genes (antibody micro-arrays) and tests for protein expression, particularly in serum, that identify differential patterns between normal patients and patients with ovarian cancer. Analysis of the presence/absence/abundance of known proteins/peptides in the serum using, Enzyme-linked ImmunoSorbent Assay (ELISA) or cytokine/antibody multiplex has yielded a number of biomarker combinations with increased specificity and sensitivity for ovarian cancer relative to CA-125 alone.[12,13] The main objective of these biomarkers is to improve clinicians' ability to accurately detect premalignant changes or early stage EOC in asymptomatic women.

After the markers are established, a major challenge is to define the right population that will benefit from the test and how to apply it in a clinical framework.

In the following sections, the authors discuss the strategies used for the development of a novel panel for the early detection of ovarian cancer, as well as the pros and cons of its clinical application.

PROTEOMICS FOR THE DETECTION OF OVARIAN CANCER

Proteomics involve the measurement of serum proteins to identify potential biomarkers.[14–17] ELISA and multiplex bead array are two main proteomic assays that have been used for the development of blood tests for early detection of ovarian cancer. These assays have yielded a number of biomarker combinations with increased specificity and sensitivity for ovarian cancer relative to CA-125 alone.[18-20] Because of the complexity and heterogeneity of ovarian cancer, no single biomarker will be able to discriminate between healthy women and ovarian cancer patients. Similarly, no single biomarker will be able to detect all subtypes and stages of the disease with a high enough specificity and sensitivity. The use of a combination of biomarker candidates would provide greater potential for early detection of ovarian cancer.[19,20] Moreover, the selection of an appropriate combination of biomarker candidates, which can be multiplexed, may provide a great potential for ovarian cancer biomarker discovery and prevalidation.

ELISA

ELISA is a biochemical technique used in immunology to detect specific proteins in a sample. It has been widely used as a diagnostic tool in medicine and involves the capture of an unknown amount of antigen onto a polystyrene microtiter plate. After antigen immobilization, it is detected using a conjugated secondary antibody, which forms a complex ("sandwich") with the antigen. The enzyme conjugated to the secondary antibody then catalyzes a reaction that yields a detectable signal. Signals are either chromogenic or fluorometric.

Multiplex Bead Array

Multiplex bead arrays permit the simultaneous quantitation of multiple proteins in solution using spectrally distinct beads coated with different antibodies. This technology allows the analysis of up to 100 different proteins in a single microplate well. Essentially, it is an ELISA on a bead. The constituents of each well are drawn up into the flow-based Luminex array reader, which identifies each specific protein/antigen based on the bead color of its corresponding antibody. This system can simultaneously quantify up to 100 protein targets in culture media, sera, or other matrices and can automatically analyze up to 96 samples in under 35 minutes. The system generates a standard curve and therefore provides specific measurements of protein concentration.[21]

DEVELOPMENT OF BIOMARKER PANELS: A ROADMAP FOR SUCCESS

A great deal of effort has been invested by multiple groups in pursuit of identifying combinations of markers that could improve the sensitivity and specificity for the diagnosis of early-stage ovarian cancer. At least 30 blood and urine markers have so far been combined with CA-125 for this purpose. These studies, however, compared only two or three markers at a time and showed an increased sensitivity but an associated decrease in specificity.

As mentioned above, for the early detection of EOC, it is crucial to develop panels of biomarkers that can increase both the sensitivity and the specificity. An ideal test should be able to distinguish between a healthy woman and a patient with early stage disease—with a high degree of specificity and sensitivity. Such a test must be reproducible, quantitative, noninvasive, and inexpensive.

The authors' approach in the development of an early detection test has followed the suggested "roadmap" proposed by Anderson and by Gagnon and Ye,[12,22] which is comprised of three phases: discovery, verification/validation, and clinical implementation. The process used in developing the final panel of protein markers involved several different screening steps, used samples obtained from different patient populations, and was validated with different techniques.

Discovery Phase

In the first step of the discovery phase, novel biomarkers were identified by comparing factors in serum or urine samples collected from healthy controls and from ovarian cancer patients. This approach seems to lead to more clinically relevant candidates, as the ultimate goal of a diagnostic test is one that is noninvasive, can be easily performed on serum or urine, and is relatively painless. In this phase, the authors used the rolling circle amplification (RCA) assay, which, like mass spectrometry, is a powerful technology for discovery but not for diagnostics. The authors first analyzed the expression levels of 169 proteins in serum samples collected from 18 untreated EOC patients and 28 healthy, age-matched controls. The authors limited the output to proteins associated with the control of cell growth and therefore avoided covering the whole proteome. In this initial screen, 35 proteins were differentially expressed between healthy women and newly diagnosed EOC patients based on ANOVA tests, with P-values of 0.05.

In the second step of the discovery phase, the authors evaluated the specificity of the 35 potential markers by changing the patient cohort. Again using the RCA technology, the authors evaluated a different patient population while maintaining the same clinical characteristics as the previous group. After further validation with an additional 40 patients, the number of potential biomarkers was reduced from 35 to 10, based on ANOVA, with P-values of less than 0.05. This second screening step has the advantage of removing potential "stress proteins" that could lead to nonspecific biomarkers. Furthermore, these results emphasize the importance of using multiple patient groups for discovery and for validation.

The third step in the discovery phase involves the evaluation of each individual marker using a different technology and preferentially one that could be used in the clinic. In this case, the authors proceeded to evaluate the markers obtained from the discovery phase using commercially available ELISA kits for each of the identified proteins.

The ELISA results showed that four proteins, out of the 10 could accurately discriminate between healthy individuals and cancer patients. These proteins were: leptin, prolactin, osteopontin (OPN) and insulin growth factor II (IGF-II). These four biomarkes showed perfect correlation between the RCA immunoassays and ELISA. In addition, the expression pattern between the control (healthy) and case (ovarian cancer) sets was different for each protein. Both prolactin and OPN were significantly elevated in EOC serum, whereas leptin and IGF-II levels were reduced.

The authors then evaluated the capacity of each protein to discriminate between the case and the control cohorts. Although each protein had an AUC significantly above 0.5, none of the markers individually had enough sensitivity and specificity. Only when used together was the panel of biomarkers able to discriminate between control and cancer group samples.

To differentiate between healthy subjects and ovarian cancer patients, and healthy subjects after sample decoding, the authors evaluated several statistical approaches and used statistical cluster analysis for the final model. First, split points for each biomarker were established. The split point divides the sample space into two intervals: one for normal and another for cancer. The best split point for each marker was chosen to minimize the number of misclassified individuals. Using split point analysis with four markers, cancer is predicted by having two or more markers in the abnormal range and a normal finding is defined by one or zero markers in the abnormal range.

Validation Phase

The first step in the validation process is the evaluation of the model in a blind study. Thus, the authors used a cohort consisting of 206 serum samples, which included samples from 106 healthy subjects and 100 ovarian cancer patients (24 stage I/II and 76 stage III/IV). The model was able to identify 96 out of 100 EOC patients (96%), including 23 of 24 patients with stage I/II EOC. In the healthy group, 6 of 106 individual were incorrectly diagnosed (5.6%).

The final results of the test have shown a sensitivity of 95% and a specificity of 95%, (**Fig. 1**). Therefore, not only did ELISA provide a platform for the quantitative measurement of proteins and assay reproducibility, there was also verification in pattern of response of biomarkers between RCA and ELISA.[19,20]

CLINICAL IMPLEMENTATION

Although ELISA could discriminate between healthy and early stage disease with a high degree of specificity and sensitivity, there are limitations with the use of this technology for a multiple biomarker test. The first limitation is the potential variability in overall results between the different ELISA kits, and second is the high cost of performing multiple ELISAs. Therefore, the use of Multiplex bead array could represent a better approach for this type of tests.

Multiplex bead array provides numerous advantages as a platform for the diagnostic implementation.[19] With Multiplex bead array, one has the ability to measure multiple markers in a small sample volume. Thus, this platform could simplify the development of a diagnostic test and could decrease the potential interassay variability. This result makes the Multiplex bead array suitable for large validation studies.

The authors' first objective was to determine whether a multiplex bead array could adequately replicate the results previously obtained with ELISA. Therefore, the authors compared concentrations obtained for prolactin, leptin, OPN and IGF-II from by ELISA and a multiplex bead array using 50 serum samples from newly diagnosed ovarian cancer patients and 50 serum samples from age-matched healthy individuals. Results showed that both ELISA and multiplex assay exhibited the same pattern for the four markers. Statistical analysis of the values obtained from the Multiplex assay showed

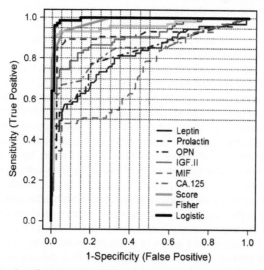

Fig. 1. Receiver Operating Characteristics (ROC) curves for composite predictors, corresponding to final model using four markers and the six markers with the different cohorts. Note the improvement with the six markers and the similarity of the results independent on the cohort analyzed.

similar results to that previously reported using ELISA (95% sensitivity and 94% specificity).

Thus, the authors selected this platform as a potential replacement for the combination ELISA; in addition, two markers were added to the panel: macrophage inhibitory factor (MIF), which was found to be highly expressed in the serum of ovarian cancer patients,[23] and CA-125. The combination of these six biomarkers is more than adequate to provide the sensitivity and specificity required but not sizable enough to impede and complicate evaluation.

The characterization of this new panel was done following the same guidelines as described for the biomarkers using ELISA. That is, a test group was used for creating the model and a different test group was used to create the model. In both steps, evaluation was done in a blind manner. The statistical results for the final model indicates a sensitivity of 95.3% and specificity of 99.4%.[24]

The multiplex bead array for the detection of ovarian cancer was developed in collaboration with Millipore. The kit, known as the Beadlyte Cancer Biomarker Panel Kit, includes two panels: one for leptin, prolactin, MIF, OPN, and CA-125 (Beadlyte 5-plex Cancer Panel); and a separate panel for IGF-II (Beadlyte Anti-human IGF-II Bead Set).

The panel is manufactured under strict regulatory conditions ensuring the reproducibility of each batch and a low coefficient of variation (intra- and inter-CV%), two important requirements for its application in clinical trials and potential clinical use.

BIOLOGICAL RELEVANCE OF THE MARKERS

The biological significance of the described biomarkers provides for a better understanding of the test. The proteins identified in this study, with the exception of CA-125 and MIF, are all related to the normal physiology of the ovaries. These proteins are produced either by the surrounding supportive cells or as a response to signals originating from the ovary. IGF-II is the primary IGF in the human ovary, acting as mediator of gonadotropin action.[25,26] Prolactin on the other hand, has been shown to participate in the regulation of steroidogenesis in ovarian follicles, particularly the inhibition of progesterone secretion in the early stages of the follicular growth and its enhancement in the luteal phase.[27,28] There is strong evidence that links leptin and the hypothalamic gonadotropin releasing hormone secretion, which affects the hypothalamic pituitary-ovarian axis.[29] Osteopontin is overexpressed in a cancers including lung cancer, breast cancer, colorectal cancer, stomach cancer, ovarian cancer, melanoma and mesothelioma.[30,31] CA-125 is a mucinous glycoprotein and product of the MUC16 gene, and a protein antigen found in abnormally high levels in the serum of women who have ovarian cancer. However, as already stated, CA-125 is not specific enough to be used for population-based screening due to its poor specificity.[13] MIF is an inflammatory mediator involved in cell-mediated immunity, immunoregulation, and inflammation.[32,33]

The level of expression of these proteins is maintained by a delicate balance between each of the cellular components of the ovary. The authors hypothesize that the presence of abnormal cells may alter this intercellular communication and disrupt the axis, resulting in the abnormal expression levels observed in cancer samples. The proteins identified in this study may not represent factors produced by the tumor but instead represent the organ/body's response to the presence of neoplastic cells. The authors propose that significant levels of products secreted by the tumor could only be detected in peripheral blood at later stages of tumor development; however, the body is able to recognize and respond to early stages of the tumorigenicity, and this is reflected in peripheral blood proteins. Based on this premise, the protein panel identified in this study is able to detect early stages of the disease.

CLINICAL APPLICATION: WHO AND WHEN

A major concern associated with the clinical use of biomarkers is the potential "false positives." The PPV is used as the standard for the determination of potential benefit/risk of the test. As indicated above, ovarian cancer is a "rare" but lethal disease. Any test, even with a specificity of 99.9%, will have a PPV not larger than 10% if it is calculated based on the general population. It means that only 1 of 10 women who were positive for the test would have ovarian cancer. If that approach is adopted, there is no value in developing a test. This is true for all forms of cancers which have a low incidence, such as ovarian and pancreatic cancer.

Based on this knowledge, there is a general consensus in the biomarker-research community that screening the general population has no value. It is, therefore, necessary to focus on specific groups where the risk of developing the cancer is higher. This population might be the group that can benefit from the test.[10]

The value of a test exists when it is applied to what is considered a high-risk population, which may further differ in incidences because of different genetic background and family history. For these cases, it is necessary to calculate PPV for each subgroup. Research on previous screening technologies suggests that cancers detected by screening may be more likely to have clinicopathologic features and better prognosis than cancers diagnosed clinically. Therefore, to obtain valid estimates of sensitivity, specificity, and predictive values for screening women at high-risk, research may need to be conducted within the specified high risk populations, not among women in the general population.

Furthermore, no blood test, in any clinical context, even with a high PPV, is meant to be used as a final diagnosis. A blood test is usually inexpensive, and it can be performed repeatedly. In the context of ovarian cancer, a blood test would provide an excellent alternative to less sensitive, more invasive, and more expensive tests such as imaging. A blood test will limit the use of CT scan or MR imaging unless clearly indicated.

Another major concern is that the use of these types of test will lead to unnecessary surgeries. Interestingly, the recommended approach for the prevention of ovarian cancer for patients in the high-risk group is preventive surgery (salpingo-oophorectomy).[34] However, from 100 preventive oophorectomies, only one or two cancers are identified.[35] Therefore, 98 women undergo unnecessary surgeries. The use of this test may help to postpone or completely avoid the surgical procedure if the results of the test are negative.

SUMMARY

This article has discussed the steps in the development and characterization of a test for detection of ovarian cancer using three different platforms, four types of statistical analysis, and two different sample cohorts. The use of this or other panels with similar sensitivity and specificity provides a potential viable alternative to screening for CA-125 alone for the diagnosis of ovarian cancer. The implementation of this test for a high-risk population may postpone or completely avoid unnecessary surgical procedures and may provide an additional tool for the management of this deadly disease.

ACKNOWLEDGMENT

These studies were supported in part by Nicolas Brady, the Adler Foundation, and the Discovery to Cure Translational Research Program.

REFERENCES

1. Permuth-Wey J, Sellers TA. Epidemiology of ovarian cancer. Methods Mol Biol 2009;472:413–37.
2. Jemal A, Siegel R, Ward E, et al. Cancer statistics, 2006. CA Cancer J Clin 2006; 56(2):106–30.
3. Schwartz PE. Current diagnosis and treatment modalities for ovarian cancer. Cancer Treat Res 2002;107:99–118.
4. Berchuck A, Elbendary A, Havrilesky L, et al. Pathogenesis of ovarian cancers. J Soc Gynecol Investig 1994;1(3):181–90.
5. Goff BA, Muntz HG. Screening and early diagnosis of ovarian cancer. Women's Health in Primary Care 2005;8(6):262–8.
6. Miller BA, Chu KC, Hankey BF, et al. Cancer incidence and mortality patterns among specific Asian and Pacific Islander populations in the U.S. Cancer Causes Control 2008;19(3):227–56.
7. Espey DK, Wu XC, Swan J, et al. Annual report to the nation on the status of cancer, 1975-2004, featuring cancer in American Indians and Alaska Natives. Cancer 2007;110(10):2119–52.
8. Mutch D. Surgical manegement of ovarian cancer. Semin Oncol 2002;29:3–8.
9. Permuth-Wey J, Boulware D, Valkov N, et al. Sampling strategies for tissue micro-arrays to evaluate biomarkers in ovarian cancer. Cancer Epidemiol Biomarkers Prev 2009;18(1):28–34.
10. Nick AM, Sood AK. The ROC 'n' role of the multiplex assay for early detection of ovarian cancer. Nat Clin Pract Oncol 2008;5(10):568–9.
11. Berger RP, Ta'asan S, Rand A, et al. Multiplex assessment of serum biomarker concentrations in well-appearing children with inflicted traumatic brain injury. Pediatr Res 2008;65:97–102.
12. Gagnon A, Ye B. Discovery and application of protein biomarkers for ovarian cancer. Curr Opin Obstet Gynecol 2008;20(1):9–13.
13. Bast RC Jr, Badgwell D, Lu Z, et al. New tumor markers: CA125 and beyond. Int J Gynecol Cancer 2005;15(Suppl 3):274–81.
14. Wu B, Abbott T, Fishman D, et al. Comparison of statistical methods for classification of ovarian cancer using mass spectrometry data. Bioinformatics 2003; 19(13):1636–43.
15. Bast RC Jr, Brewer M, Zou C, et al. Prevention and early detection of ovarian cancer: mission impossible? Recent Results Cancer Res 2007;174:91–100.
16. Petricoin EF, Ardekani AM, Hitt BA, et al. Use of proteomic patterns in serum to identify ovarian cancer. Lancet 2002;359(9306):572–7.
17. Chang J, Powles TJ, Allred DC, et al. Biologic markers as predictors of clinical outcome from systemic therapy for primary operable breast cancer. J Clin Oncol 1999;17(10):3058–63.
18. Woolas RP, Xu FJ, Jacobs IJ, et al. Elevation of multiple serum markers in patients with stage I ovarian cancer. J Natl Cancer Inst 1993;85(21):1748–51.
19. Gorelik E, Landsittel DP, Marrangoni AM, et al. Multiplexed immunobead-based cytokine profiling for early detection of ovarian cancer. Cancer Epidemiol Biomarkers Prev 2005;14(4):981–7.
20. Mor G, Visintin I, Lai Y, et al. Serum protein markers for early detection of ovarian cancer. Proc Natl Acad Sci U S A 2005;102(21):7677–82.
21. Vignali DA. Multiplexed particle-based flow cytometric assays. J Immunol Methods 2000;243(1–2):243–55.

22. Anderson NL. The roles of multiple proteomic platforms in a pipeline for new diagnostics. Mol Cell Proteomics 2005;4(10):1441–4.
23. Agarwal R, Alvero A, Visintin I, et al. Macrophage migration inhibitory factor expression in ovarian cancer. Am J Obstet Gynecol 2007;196(4):348.e1–5.
24. Visintin I, Feng Z, Longton G, et al. Diagnostic markers for early detection of ovarian cancer. Clin Cancer Res 2008;14(4):1065–72.
25. Giudice LC. Insulin-like growth factor family in Graafian follicle development and function. J Soc Gynecol Investig 2001;8(1 Suppl Proceedings):S26–9.
26. Kaipia A, Hsueh AJ. Regulation of ovarian follicle atresia. Annu Rev Physiol 1997; 59:349–63.
27. Grosdemouge I, Bachelot A, Lucas A, et al. Effects of deletion of the prolactin receptor on ovarian gene expression. Reprod Biol Endocrinol 2003;1–12.
28. Bachelot A, Binart N. Corpus luteum development: lessons from genetic models in mice. Curr Top Dev Biol 2005;68:49–84.
29. Popovic V, Casanueva FF. Leptin, nutrition and reproduction: new insights. Hormones (Athens) 2002;1(4):204–17.
30. Brakora KA, Lee H, Yusuf R, et al. Utility of osteopontin as a biomarker in recurrent epithelial ovarian cancer. Gynecol Oncol 2004;93(2):361–5.
31. Chambers AF, Vanderhyden BC. Ovarian cancer biomarkers in urine. Clin Cancer Res 2006;12(2):323–7.
32. Morand EF, Leech M, Weedon H, et al. Macrophage migration inhibitory factor in rheumatoid arthritis: clinical correlations. Rheumatology (Oxford) 2002;41(5): 558–62.
33. Mitchell RA, Liao H, Chesney J, et al. Macrophage migration inhibitory factor (MIF) sustains macrophage proinflammatory function by inhibiting p53: regulatory role in the innate immune response. Proc Natl Acad Sci U S A 2002;99(1): 345–50.
34. Piver MS, Jishi MF, Tsukada Y, et al. Primary peritoneal carcinoma after prophylactic oophorectomy in women with a family history of ovarian cancer. A report of the Gilda Radner Familial Ovarian Cancer Registry. Cancer 1993;71(9):2751–5.
35. Finch A, Beiner M, Lubinski J, et al. Salpingo-oophorectomy and the risk of ovarian, fallopian tube, and peritoneal cancers in women with a BRCA1 or BRCA2 mutation. JAMA 2006;296(2):185–92.

Analytical Considerations for Mass Spectrometry Profiling in Serum Biomarker Discovery

Gordon R. Whiteley, PhD, MSc[a,*], Simona Colantonio, MPharm, PhD[a,b], Andrea Sacconi, DEng[a,b], Richard G. Saul, PhD, BS[a]

KEYWORDS

- Biomarkers • Proteomic patterns • MALDI
- Bioinformatics • Reproducibility • Immune Capture
- Carrier proteins • Low molecular weight proteome

The potential of mass spectrometry patterns as a diagnostic tool was first described in 2002 and was hailed as a breakthrough in diagnostic medicine.[1] Although this first report was a concept paper, many interpreted it as a completed test ready for commercialization. A resulting storm of controversy criticizing the concept was based largely on theoretical concerns.[2,3] At the same time, proteomic patterns for a long list of additional diseases were reported[4–6] and the debate continued. Indeed, there are still reports of proteomic patterns that are being discovered for diseases but with a heavy focus on early cancer detection.[7,8] There was and still is a lack of focus on the development of a method that is well understood and controlled and could be used in a clinical study to determine the true feasibility of this technology as a diagnostic tool. There are, however, several breakthroughs both in the understanding of proteomic patterns from the laboratory testing of samples and in the bioinformatics

This project has been funded in whole or in part with federal funds from the National Cancer Institute, National Institutes of Health, under contract number N01-CO-12,400. The content of this publication does not necessarily reflect the views or policies of the Department of Health and Human Services, nor does mention of trade names, commercial products, or organizations imply endorsement by the US Government. This research was supported in part by the Developmental Therapeutics Program in the Division of Cancer Treatment and Diagnosis of the National Cancer Institute.

[a] Clinical Proteomics Reference Lab, Advanced Technology Program, SAIC-Frederick, NCI-Frederick, PO Box B, Frederick, MD 21702, USA
[b] Department of Molecular Medicine, "Regina Elena" National Cancer Institute, Rome, Via Elio Chianersi, 53, 00144 Rome, Italy
* Corresponding author.
E-mail address: WhiteleyG@ncifcrf.gov (G.R. Whiteley).

Clin Lab Med 29 (2009) 57–69
doi:10.1016/j.cll.2009.01.003
0272-2712/09/$ – see front matter © 2009 Elsevier Inc. All rights reserved.

labmed.theclinics.com

analysis that will result in clinically useful information for diagnosis and further understanding of the disease process.

THE ROLE OF SURFACE-ENHANCED LASER DESORPTION IONIZATION SYSTEM IN PROTEOMICS AWARENESS

The term "proteomics" first appeared in the early 1990s but did not become common in the scientific literature until much later in that decade.[9] At about the same time, the surface-enhanced laser desorption ionization (SELDI) system was introduced by Ciphergen (Fremont, California, now called BioRad). This technique was a fusion of sample fractionation and matrix-assisted laser desorption ionization (MALDI) mass spectrometry. The company had made both the sample preparation and instrumentation simple to use and convenient for processing large numbers of samples. For the first time, it was possible for scientists in the biologic sciences to investigate mass spectrometry in their laboratories without having to tackle the complexities of the other mass spectrometer instruments available. The SELDI arrays were designed with an increased surface area within a series of eight circles surrounded by a hydrophobic membrane (**Fig. 1**). Samples were processed on 12 arrays that were held in a device that gave the standard 96 configuration of a 96-well microtiter plate. This allowed for high throughput processing and adaptation to robotic platforms designed for ELISA tests. The arrays were then read by the compact (for that time) mass spectrometer instrument. A user-friendly software gave presentation of results in formats familiar to biologists, such as the "gel view" graphic representation of spectra in a density plot.[1,10]

In a groundbreaking report, Petricoin and colleagues[1] reported the use of this system to test a group of ovarian cancer patient samples and a group of samples that were free of ovarian cancer. Once the spectra had been collected from the sample sets, a genetic algorithm and self-organizing cluster analysis was used to find differences in the spectral patterns between the two groups. Masked samples were then used to test the discovered patterns and the results gave a startling sensitivity and

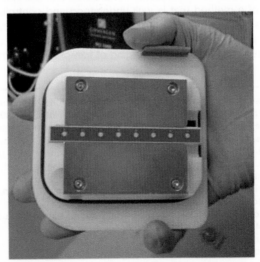

Fig. 1. The SELDI array consisting of eight spots (silver) surrounded by a hydrophobic membrane (brown). Twelve of these arrays can be held together in a configuration that has the footprint of a microtiter plate.

specificity of 100% and 95%, respectively. This report was followed rapidly by reports from many authors finding patterns for other cancers and diseases and new patterns are being reported even now.[7,8,11-13]

SURFACE-ENHANCED LASER DESORPTION IONIZATION SYSTEM GOES HIGH RESOLUTION

One of the disadvantages of the SELDI system is that the resolution is not sufficient for identification of peptides. This was overcome when Ciphergen produced a SELDI front-end to a high-resolution instrument, the ABI Q-star. It allowed the SELDI arrays to be read with higher resolution but the throughput was low and did not allow for large sample sets to be easily processed. As biologists became more comfortable with mass spectrometry, profiling was evaluated on this platform with results that seemed to be absolutely accurate compared with the original results found on the Ciphergen instrumentation (**Table 1**).[14] There were a total of four models that gave 100% sensitivity and specificity but it was noted that there were several peaks common to all of the algorithms that gave high-accuracy results. As both excitement and criticism grew over the possibility of using this technology for early detection of cancer and other diseases, the need for evaluation of reproducibility, robustness, control, and understanding of the mechanism of the method became more urgent.

PRINCIPLE OF THE TEST

The most fundamental issue before dealing with reproducibility and robustness was the question of the principle of the test and what exactly was being measured. What was curious in the initial reports was that the potential biomarkers being measured could be detected by a mass spectrometer whose sensitivity is some two orders of magnitude less than the standard ELISA technique (Richard G. Saul and Gordon R. Whiteley, unpublished data, 2005). It just did not seem possible to measure products of small primary stage tumors in the large volume of plasma using this technique. This was soon explained, however, by the possibility that biomarkers were being collected and concentrated in the serum by high-abundance carrier proteins, such as albumin.[15] Albumin is known to be a carrier protein and one with a relatively long half-life of 19 days.[16] Traditional mass spectrometry concentrated on the removal of the high-abundance proteins to detect the low concentration peptides and proteins in serum hoping that these would yield biomarkers for disease. The revolutionary thought that the biomarkers may indeed be discarded with the removal of the carrier proteins, however, led to the discovery that there were ion species correlating with cancer, such as ovarian cancer associated with these carrier proteins. By isolating the albumin and then dissociating low-molecular-weight peptides and proteins, a further large number of cancer-related proteins and peptides along with new unique peptides were also found.[17] This discovery was instrumental in the development and approach of other studies that have since shown patterns of albumin-associated peptides for Alzheimer's disease,[13] ovarian cancer,[18] cutaneous T-cell lymphoma,[19] and breast cancer.[20] It has also provided the basis for the isolation and concentration of peptides that are now being studied as potential biomarkers.

AUTOMATION OF THE PROCESS

One of the earliest tools for making the SELDI and other MALDI platforms more robust was automation of sample preparation, thereby eliminating bias introduced by person-to-person technique variability. Early in the proteomic profiling studies using the Ciphergen system, automation was a key to both ease of high throughput processing

Table 1
Four computer models that identified test sets of samples with ovarian cancer with a sensitivity and specificity of 100%

Model 1			Model 2		
Test specificity		100%	Test specificity		100%
Test sensitivity		100%	Test sensitivity		100%
Validation specificity		100%	Validation specificity		100%
Validation sensitivity		100%	Validation sensitivity		100%
Result breakdown			Result breakdown		
State	Testing results (%)	Validation results (%)	State	Testing results (%)	Validation results (%)
Normal	30/30 (100)	37/37 (100)	Normal	31/31 (100)	37/37 (100)
Ovarian cancer	57/57 (100)	40/40 (100)	Ovarian cancer	63/63 (100)	40/40 (100)
Stage 1	17/17 (100)	12/12 (100)	Stage 1	22/22 (100)	12/12 (100)
Distinguishing m/z values			Distinguishing m/z values		
1 1276.8612			1 818.4801		
2 2374.2444			2 6352.7227		
3 4292.9			3 6548.771		
4 7060.121			4 7060.121		
5 8605.678			5 7096.9224		
6 8706.065			6 8540.536		
7 9870.9375			7 8605.678		
8 —			8 8706.065		
Model 3			**Model 4**		
Test specificity		100%	Test specificity		100%
Test sensitivity		100%	Test sensitivity		100%
Validation specificity		100%	Validation specificity		100%
Validation sensitivity		100%	Validation sensitivity		100%
Result breakdown			Result breakdown		
State	Testing results (%)	Validation results (%)	State	Testing results (%)	Validation results (%)
Normal	31/31 (100)	37/37 (100)	Normal	31/31 (100)	37/37 (100)
Ovarian cancer	63/63 (100)	40/40 (100)	Ovarian cancer	63/63 (100)	40/40 (100)
Stage 1	22/22 (100)	12/12 (100)	Stage 1	22/22 (100)	12/12 (100)
Distinguishing m/z values			Distinguishing m/z values		
1 1144.7963			1 1001.6544		
2 4260.4033			2 1255.5934		
3 7046.018			3 4377.8535		
4 8602.237			4 6004.4165		
5 8664.385			5 7060.121		
6 —			6 7202.716		
7 —			7 8605.678		
8 —			8 8709.548		
9 —			9 9367.113		

Note the repeating ions that appear in more than one of the models.

Adapted from Conrads TP, Fusaro VA, Ross S, et al. High-resolution serum proteomic features for ovarian cancer detection. Endocr Relat Cancer 2004;11:163; with permission.

and reproducibility. The Beckman Biomek system was originally packaged with the Ciphergen system and sold as part of the system. This microplate processor platform was easy to program and the design of the 96-spot microplate layout made the adaptation of the system simple. It was observed, however, that the matrix application timing was critical to reproducibility and this observation was confirmed by others.[21] Furthermore, it was found that the drying time of the sample on the arrays was also critical and this finding was also observed by others.[22] These factors needed to be taken into account when selecting a robotics system.

The weak point of the original Biomek system was that the matrix application was done one spot at a time and it took close to 1 hour to apply matrix to all 96 positions. The Tecan Genesis system (Tecan AG, Switzerland) was later converted and a system of serpentine matrix application was programmed that substantially reduced the application time. This along with the installation of the robot in a laboratory that was both temperature ($\pm$ 2°C) and humidity ($\pm$ 5%) controlled led to an improvement in the robustness of the technology.[20] The final adaptation to robotic processing was done using the Hamilton Star robot (Hamilton, Reno, Nevada). This robot uses a unique method to pick up pipette tips and has a 96-head pipettor capable of application of 1 μL of matrix to all positions with great precision. That allowed the simultaneous application of matrix and eliminated the matrix addition timing as a potential source of variability. This robot became the basis for both SELDI and MALDI studies done within the authors' laboratory.[19,23,24]

REPRODUCIBILITY AND ROBUSTNESS FACTORS

Although the adaptation of sample processing was an important factor in stabilizing reproducibility, it was only one of many factors that were keys. Indeed, many of the top-level requirements were outlined in an editorial in 2005 (**Box 1**).[25] This sobering reality brought attention beyond the analytical platform to issues of sample acquisition and handling along with the data processing, both critical components of technology robustness.

The influence of presampling factors on the human proteomic pattern has not been thoroughly studied. There are studies emerging on the manipulation of the proteome through such factors as diet in fish[26] and rats[27] with the expected result that there are changes in the proteome induced by dietary changes. Some of the identified proteins involved are apolipoprotein A and aldolase, both of which have been identified as potential sentinels of disease.[28] One can also assume that other factors, such as medication, diet, and hormonal status, could disrupt the human proteome and must be either accounted for or diluted out in studies of disease through proteomic patterns.[29] The careful selection of patient populations becomes a critical part of these studies, especially during the validation of any proteomic pattern.[30]

The next set of issues involves the acquisition, handling, and processing of samples before testing. There are some studies that have been done on these various aspects but no standard procedure has been set. A comparison of serum and plasma as sources demonstrated expected differences in the two samples.[31] It was also observed by Banks and colleagues[31] that there was significant alteration of the profiles when there was a delay in the time between sample acquisition and processing. Clotting time for serum was found to be significant and it was suggested that a time greater than 30 minutes was necessary for all of the changes resulting from clotting to be at a steady state. There has also been an observation that the many possible additives to tubes show potential for differences in observed ions[32] and the only tubes that seemed to be suitable for serum were glass tubes without additives. Storage is another issue.[33]

Box 1
Recommended practices for clinical applications of protein profiling by matrix-assisted laser desorption and ionization time of-flight mass spectrometry

Preanalytical

- Evaluate optimum patient preparation
- Identify optimum procedures for specimen collection and processing
- Analyze specimen stability
- Develop criteria for specimen acceptability

Analytical

- Prepare calibrators for mass, resolution, and detector sensitivity
- Use internal standards
- Automate specimen preparation
- Optimize methods to yield highest possible signals for peaks of interest
- Identify sequences of peaks of interest
- Develop calibration materials for components of interest
- Quality control: prepare and identify at least two concentrations of control material
- Evaluate reproducibility (precision)
- Evaluate limits of detection and linearity
- Evaluate reference intervals
- Evaluate interferences, such as hemolysis, lipemia, renal failure, acute-phase responses
- Develop materials or programs for external comparison and proficiency testing of analyzers

Postanalytical

- Analyze each spectrum to identify peaks before applying diagnostic algorithms
- Develop criteria for the acceptability of each spectrum based on peak characteristics
- Use peaks rather than raw data as the basis for diagnostic analysis
- Use caution in interpretation of peaks with mass/charge <1200
- Select peaks with high intensities and sample stability for diagnosis
- Select approximately equal numbers of peaks that increase and decrease in intensity as diagnostic discriminators
- In developing a training set for diagnosis, careful clinical classification of patients is essential
- Clinical validity depends on having a typical rather than highly selected population of patients
- The number of training specimens should be at least 10 times the number of measured values
- Any clinical application should use a fixed training set and algorithm for analysis
- Any analysis should provide a numerical value
- Diagnostic performance should be evaluated with receiver operating characteristic curves to select cutoffs
- A sensitivity analysis should be performed of the necessary precision for accurate diagnostic performance
- There should be quality control procedures for daily verification of software performance

Adapted from Hortin GL. Can mass spectrometric protein profiling meet desired standards of clinical laboratory practice? Clin Chem 2005;51:3; with permission.

Freezing was shown not to impact the patterns.[34] It was also found that freezing and thawing did not impact the patterns. Samples stored at 2°C to 8°C, however, did show a significant drop in the area of the spectra around the 3800 to 4000 m/z range (W.B. Shand and Gordon R. Whiteley, unpublished data, October 2006). Additional studies done in animals also demonstrated the issues of sample handling and processing and their impact on spectra.[35]

Sample preparation for mass spectrometry can have yet a further impact on the spectra. It was found that temperature and humidity were critical issues for the drying of samples and matrix[20] and these findings were confirmed in a more formal study.[34] The influence of pH, buffer concentration, and surface selected can also cause shifts in proteomic pattern[2] and these can be misinterpreted as lack of reproducibility.[36] What is clear is that there needs to be definition of not only the factors that can influence reproducibility but also the limitations of each of these factors. Controls or indicators of these factors can assist researchers in guiding data interpretation so that patterns can be reliably reproduced.

DEMONSTRATIONS OF REPRODUCIBILITY

Despite all of these issues, there have been very promising demonstrations of the power and reproducibility of proteomic patterns. The earliest comprehensive report appeared in 2005 where six sites were asked to prepare and test samples using a standard protocol after a rigorous calibration with known proteins (insulin and IgG), a standardized pooled sample. Known peaks were evaluated for intensity, resolution, and signal-to-noise ratio. After this, sites were asked to test 14 prostate cancer and 14 noncancer samples and analyze the data using a standardized method. Their results showed that, under these conditions, they were able to show agreement between laboratories to a high degree of confidence.[37] Another study demonstrated reproducibility of a pattern for breast cancer over a 14-month period using the same instrumentation, method, and highly controlled conditions.[20] This was the first time that the potential of patterns being stable over time had been reported. Within-patient stability of profiles has also been demonstrated.[38] In this study, individual patient samples taken over a 3-year period were examined. Although some peaks showed high coefficient of variation values, the authors concluded that there were sufficient peaks with good reproducibility that the spectra from this group of patients were stable. It should be noted, however, that these samples were all run at the same time, reducing the issues regarding control of the sample processing and instrumentation listed previously.

THE USE OF BIOINFORMATICS TO FIND PATTERNS

The complexity of mass spectra compounded with a significant number of samples within each of a "training group" dictates that sophisticated computer analysis methods be used to find patterns that correlate with disease. Most of the techniques used were originally designed for other purposes involving pattern recognition to extract information from surveillance and other data. The first mass spectrometry patterns were revealed with the use of genetic algorithms and self-organizing maps.[1] Since that time, a number of programs have been developed by mass spectrometry manufacturers, such as the Cipergen Biomarker Wizard software. An earlier version of this software was used to identify biomarkers for ovarian cancer[39] and these are the basis for a series of markers now in clinical evaluations by Vermillion that has been filed with the Food and Drug Administration (http://ir.ciphergen.com/preview/phoenix.zhtml?c=121814&p=irol-newsArticle&ID=1169372&highlight=). The same types of software have also been used in the world of genetic analysis to reveal gene patterns that are indicative of disease.[40]

Mass spectra are so complex, however, that before analysis there must be some processing of the data. This involves the separation of true signal from noise that can be the result of both chemical and spectral baseline noise. Each of these can in themselves cause problems with the data analysis unless particular care is taken. One of the great assets of mass spectral data is its high dimensionality, but this is also one of the great issues in efficient data mining. To reduce the dimensionality, binning of data is usually done. This can be done by the addition of peaks at fixed distances along the spectrum but is much better performed when the data are binned in a growing window taking advantage of the higher resolution of instruments at the lower mass-charge (m/z) range and compensating for the lower resolution at the high m/z end of the spectrum. Algorithms for binning have also been developed using only areas between two valleys in the spectrum.[19] This method helps preserve peaks and avoid loss of resolution caused by the accidental addition of separate peaks because of their location within a fixed m/z range. Once this is done, pattern analysis can be performed.

The authors' approach has been to simplify or have redundant analysis as much as possible to have confidence in patterns that were observed to avoid the pitfalls of each of the methods that are well documented. The method is described in detail in the publication by Liu and colleagues.[19] Briefly, peaks that showed significant intensity differences between disease and nondisease groups were selected. Then three classification methods were used: (1) partial least square regression, (2) support vector machine, and (3) the C5.0 decision tree. Each of the test samples were classified by the three methods and then a voting scheme was used for the final classification. Where disagreement occurred, the samples were classified as unknown. The classification showed that complex patterns existed showing differences between these two groups. A simpler approach, however, took advantage of the true power of mass spectrometry: the ability to detect very small differences in a molecule caused by a posttranslational modification. Using this method, an algorithm of peak pair ratios selected peak pairs correlating with posttranslational modifications associated with cancer that showed significant differences between patients with ovarian cancer and patients without disease. The result was that four peak pairs (eight peaks) could differentiate between these two groups in a test group of samples. This finding showed that there were potential biomarkers of disease markers to be discovered in these samples.

PROTEOMIC PATTERNS AS POTENTIAL DIAGNOSTIC TOOLS

This seems to be extremely challenging and will probably require significant breakthroughs in all areas: mass spectrometry, computer software, understanding of sample issues, and methods of controlling all aspects of testing. Despite this, the authors did assess the feasibility of the technology using a set of patient samples and the previously mentioned developed algorithm. The original algorithm was developed from samples collected at Northwestern University under their protocol. Samples were stored at $-80°C$ until testing. A set of blinded samples were collected and processed at a second institution (Duke University). There was no review of the sample collection and processing protocol to make it consistent with that of Northwestern University. The samples were also frozen at $-80°C$ before testing. The method for sample preparation and testing was consistent in the laboratory and all tests were done on the same instrumentation under the same conditions. The spectra were processed and classified according to the previously mentioned algorithm. The final results had been blinded up until this point. The results showed that there was a significant agreement between the classification and clinical diagnosis when unblinded, although the sensitivity and specificity were much lower than in the test group and there were a significant number of samples classified as unknown (**Table 2**). Although this clearly shows that the methodology needs substantial development before it can be used in a clinical trial, it demonstrates that there are potential biomarkers that should be investigated.

GUIDED BIOMARKER DISCOVERY USING PROTEOMIC PATTERNS

Once a pattern has been found, it is not a trivial task to identify the proteins that are the source of the pattern. Using high-resolution MALDI results such as those obtained previously, however, it is conceivable to sort through the spectra of the sample collection and select individual samples with high intensities of the peaks of interest and samples with extremely low intensities of these same peaks. Using these samples, the process of fractionation and the search for the identity begins with the knowledge that the MALDI database identification can confirm a more definitive methodology.

Several methods have been successfully used to identify proteins. These include conventional chemical methods, such as Edman's degradation, but the more sophisticated and less laborious mass spectrometry techniques are now more commonly used. Both high-resolution platforms used in MALDI experiments and tandem mass spectrometry are significant tools in the identification process. The MALDI TOF-TOF platform measures the mass-charge value with extremely high-resolution through a double time of flight configuration essentially magnifying the scale on which values are plotted.[41] The tandem mass spectrometry platforms provide for ion fragmentation giving multiple daughter ions. These are then measured and the identification can be done with more confidence based on multiple ions resulting from each observed parent ion.[42] For complex mixtures, such as serum, a fractionation is done that mimics the fractionation done before the original spectral patterns are generated. This is then followed by further fractionations to reduce the complexity of the samples. These fractionations can be done using such methods as electrophoresis (either one or two dimensional) or liquid chromatography followed by mass spectrometry on either digested fragments or the intact material. Identification is then done using database searching and sophisticated software to match the observed spectra with stored spectra of known proteins and peptides. This process is difficult with variable

Table 2
Classification of blinded samples from study site 2 using a classification system derived from samples collected at study site 1

	Classification		
	Normal	Cancer	Unknown
Clinical diagnosis			
Normal N = 30	23	2	5
Cancer N = 29	4	20	5

Sensitivity, 83%; specificity, 92%.
Classification was done using the peak pair algorithm and involved four peak pairs (eight peaks total).[19] Note the high number of "unknown" results.

confidence in results. Once a potential identification is made, however, other methods, such as affinity capture methods, can be used to confirm the results.

DEPLOYMENT OF PATTERNS INTO THE CLINICAL LABORATORY

The migration of this technology to the clinical environment is not an easy task. There are, however, several possibilities that could accommodate the knowledge gained by these studies and merge them with technology that is currently accepted or could be adapted to the clinical laboratory environment. The immunoassay in its many forms is a well-understood and accepted platform for clinical sample testing. Such techniques as the ELISA have exquisite sensitivity. They do not, however, have the capability of easily and accurately detecting small changes in molecules that are possible markers of disease. Mass spectrometry has the capacity to detect these very minor changes but lacks the sensitivity of the immunoassay techniques. It is logical to explore the fusion of these techniques.

Exploration of the affinity concentration and mass spectrometry techniques has been done as a way of biomarker definition and discovery. Several different solid

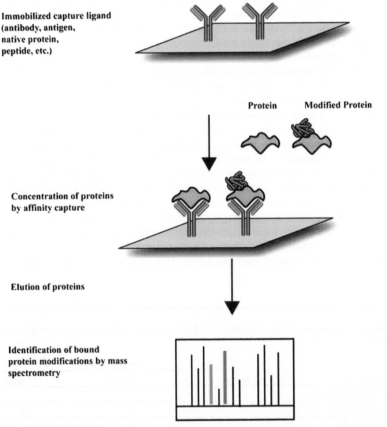

Fig. 2. Immunocapture of proteins from more complex solutions followed by the analysis of the captured material by MALDI mass spectrometry. The mass spectrometry can be done directly on the same surface or in a more concentrated fashion by elution of the captured material.

phases have been used in a basic scheme as outlined in **Fig. 2**. These have included magnetic beads,[43] affinity pipette tips,[44] and gold surfaces.[45] In each case, antibodies were used as affinity capture reagents to fractionate and concentrate proteins and peptides from more complex solutions. In the case of the magnetic beads and affinity pipette tips, the process was automated on a robotic system and proteins captured by the antibodies were eluted and analyzed by mass spectrometry. The results show that these two techniques together are powerful and provide an information-rich output that not only shows different isoforms of proteins but also quantitative information.

The use of gold surfaces adds yet another dimension.[45,46] This allows for the label-free detection of proteins captured through surface plasmon resonance, and then using the same surface the proteins can be encapsulated in matrix and MALDI mass spectrometry interrogation can be performed. Samples can be tested to see if they contain a particular binding partner to the affinity surface and then the form of the protein can be determined by mass spectrometry. The sensitivity of surface plasmon resonance is somewhat less than more sensitive amplification methods. This type of hybrid technology increases the value of the data collected through the addition of another dimension of separation and detection.

SUMMARY

Mass spectrometry patterns are a rich source of potential biomarkers for a wide variety of diseases. Although they have been described more than 5 years ago, the understanding of the source of the patterns and the identity of most of the proteins remains largely unknown. The host of factors that must be considered when using these patterns for biomarker discovery or potential diagnostic testing is extensive and still largely unexplored. The enormous potential, however, for this technology in both discovery and early diagnosis is clear. The path forward requires a tremendous amount of development work and careful clinical validation. The promise of new insight into disease mechanisms and early detection using the technique or hybrid forms with other synergistic technologies calls for additional time and effort that will result in positive patient benefit.

REFERENCES

1. Petricoin EF, Ardekani AM, Hitt BA, et al. Use of proteomic patterns in serum to identify ovarian cancer. Lancet 2002;359:572–7.
2. Baggerly KA, Morris JS, Coombes KR. Reproducibility of SELDI-TOF protein patterns in serum: comparing datasets from different experiments. Bioinformatics 2004;20:777–85.
3. Diamandis EP. Analysis of serum proteomic patterns for early cancer diagnosis: drawing attention to potential problems. J Natl Cancer Inst 2004;96:353–6.
4. Bhattacharyya S, Siegel ER, Petersen GM, et al. Diagnosis of pancreatic cancer using serum proteomic profiling. Neoplasia 2004;6:674–86.
5. Grizzle WE, Adam BL, Bigbee WL, et al. Serum protein expression profiling for cancer detection: validation of a SELDI-based approach for prostate cancer. Dis Markers 2003;19:185–95.
6. Whiteley GR. Proteomic patterns for cancer diagnosis-promise and challenges. Mol Biosyst 2006;2:358–63.
7. Wang J, Zhang X, Ge X, et al. Proteomic studies of early-stage and advanced ovarian cancer patients. Gynecol Oncol 2008;111:111–9.
8. Wei YS, Zheng YH, Liang WB, et al. Identification of serum biomarkers for nasopharyngeal carcinoma by proteomic analysis. Cancer 2008;112:544–51.

9. Abbott G. Proteomics, transcriptomics; what's in a name? Nature 1999;202: 715–6.
10. von Eggeling F, Junker K, Fiedle W, et al. Mass spectrometry meets chip technology: a new proteomic tool in cancer research? Electrophoresis 2001;22: 2898–902.
11. Adam BL, Qu Y, Davis JW, et al. Serum protein fingerprinting coupled with a pattern-matching algorithm distinguishes prostate cancer from benign prostate hyperplasia and healthy men. Cancer Res 2002;62:3609–14.
12. Honda K, Hayashida Y, Umaki T, et al. Possible detection of pancreatic cancer by plasma protein profiling. Cancer Res 2005;65:10613–22.
13. Lopez MF, Mikulskis A, Kuzdzal S, et al. High-resolution serum proteomic profiling of Alzheimer disease samples reveals disease-specific, carrier-protein-bound mass signatures. Clin Chem 2005;51:1946–54.
14. Conrads TP, Fusaro VA, Ross S, et al. High-resolution serum proteomic features for ovarian cancer detection. Endocr Relat Cancer 2004;11:163–78.
15. Mehta AI, Ross S, Lowenthal MS, et al. Biomarker amplification by serum carrier protein binding. Dis Markers 2003;19:1–10.
16. Liotta LA, Ferrari M, Petricoin E. Clinical proteomics: written in blood. Nature 2003;425:905.
17. Lowenthal MS, Mehta AI, Frogale K, et al. Analysis of albumin-associated peptides and proteins from ovarian cancer patients. Clin Chem 2005;51:1933–45.
18. Lopez MF, Mikulskis A, Kuzdzal S, et al. A novel, high-throughput workflow for discovery and identification of serum carrier protein-bound peptide biomarker candidates in ovarian cancer samples. Clin Chem 2007;53:1067–74.
19. Liu C, Shea N, Rucker S, et al. Proteomic patterns for classification of ovarian cancer and CTCL serum samples utilizing peak pairs indicative of post-translational modifications. Proteomics 2007;7:4045–52.
20. Belluco C, Petricoin EF, Mammano E, et al. Serum proteomic analysis identifies a highly sensitive and specific discriminatory pattern in stage 1 breast cancer. Ann Surg Oncol 2007;9:2470–6.
21. Jock CA, Paulauskis JD, Baker D, et al. Influence of matrix application timing on spectral reproducibility and quality in SELDI-TOF-MS. Biotechniques 2004;37: 30–2.
22. Aivado M, Spentzos D, Alterovitz G, et al. Optimization and evaluation of surface-enhanced laser desorption/ionization time-of-flight mass spectrometry (SELDI-TOF MS) with reversed-phase protein arrays for protein profiling. Clin Chem Lab Med 2005;43:133–40.
23. Cowen EW, Liu C, Steinberg SM, et al. Differentiation of tumor-phase mycosis fungoides, psoriasis vulgaris, and normal controls in a pilot study using serum proteomic analysis. Br J Dermatol 2007;22:4045–52.
24. Saul R, Russo P, Seminara S, et al. Development of an automated, mass spec-based clinical diagnostic system for the detection of ovarian cancer, Abstract WP073. Abstracts. San Jose: ALA Lab Automation Meeting; January 30–February 3, 2005. p. 205.
25. Hortin GL. Can mass spectrometric protein profiling meet desired standards of clinical laboratory practice? Clin Chem 2005;51:3–5.
26. Martin SA, Vilhelmsson O, Medale F, et al. Proteomic sensitivity to dietary manipulations in rainbow trout. Biochim Biophys Acta 2003;1651:17–29.
27. Santos-Gonzalez M, Gomez Diaz C, Navas P, et al. Modifications of plasma proteome in long-lived rats fed on a coenzyme Q10-supplemented diet. Exp Gerontol 2007;42:798–806.

28. Anderson NL, Polanski M, Pieper R, et al. The human plasma proteome: a nonredundant list developed by combination of four separate sources. Mol Cell Proteomics 2004;3:311–26.
29. Rifai N, Gillette MA, Carr SA. Protein biomarker discovery and validation: the long and uncertain path to clinical utility. Nat Biotechnol 2006;24:971–83.
30. Banks RE. Preanalytical influences in clinical proteomic studies: raising awareness of fundamental issues in sample banking. Clin Chem 2008;54:6–7.
31. Banks RE, Stanley AJ, Cairns DA, et al. Influences of blood sample processing on low-molecular-weight proteome identified by surface-enhanced laser desorption/ionization mass spectrometry. Clin Chem 2005;51:1637–49.
32. Drake SK, Bowen RA, Remaley AT, et al. Potential interferences from blood collection tubes in mass spectrometric analyses of serum polypeptides. Clin Chem 2004;50:2398–401.
33. McLerran D, Grizzle WE, Feng Z, et al. Analytical validation of serum proteomic profiling for diagnosis of prostate cancer: sources of sample bias. Clin Chem 2008;54:44–52.
34. West-Nielsen M, Hogdall EV, Marchiori E, et al. Sample handling for mass spectrometric proteomic investigations of human sera. Anal Chem 2005;77:5114–23.
35. Zhong L, Taylor DL, Whittington RJ. Proteomic profiling of ovine serum by SELDI-TOF MS: optimisation, reproducibility and feasibility of biomarker discovery using routinely collected samples. Comp Immunol Microbiol Infect Dis 2008, in press.
36. Liotta LA, Lowenthal M, Mehta A, et al. Importance of communication between producers and consumers of publicly available experimental data. J Natl Cancer Inst 2005;97:310–4.
37. Semmes OJ, Feng Z, Adam BL, et al. Evaluation of serum protein profiling by surface-enhanced laser desorption/ionization time-of-flight mass spectrometry for the detection of prostate cancer: I. Assessment of platform reproducibility. Clin Chem 2005;51:102–12.
38. Tworoger SS, Spentzos D, Grall FT, et al. Reproducibility of proteomic profiles over 3 years in postmenopausal women not taking postmenopausal hormones. Cancer Epidemiol Biomarkers Prev 2008;17:1480–5.
39. Rai AJ, Zhang Z, Rosenzweig J, et al. Proteomic approaches to tumor marker discovery. Arch Pathol Lab Med 2002;126:1518–26.
40. Whiteley G. Bringing diagnostic technologies to the clinical lab: rigor, regulation and reality. Proteomics 2008;2:1378–85.
41. Hillenkamp F, Peter-Kataliniâc J. MALDI MS: a practical guide to instrumentation, methods and applications. Weinheim (Germany): Wiley-VCH; 2007. p. 384.
42. Ducret A, Van Oostveen I, Eng JK, et al. High throughput protein characterization by automated reverse-phase chromatography/electrospray tandem mass spectrometry. Protein Sci 1998;7:706–19.
43. Whiteaker JR, Zhao L, Zhang HY, et al. Antibody-based enrichment of peptides on magnetic beads for mass-spectrometry-based quantification of serum biomarkers. Anal Biochem 2007;362:44–54.
44. Nedelkov D. Mass spectrometry-based immunoassays for the next phase of clinical applications. Expert Rev Proteomics 2006;3:631–40.
45. Nedelkov D. Development of surface plasmon resonance mass spectrometry array platform. Anal Chem 2007;79:5987–90.
46. Nedelkov D, Nelson RW. Surface plasmon resonance mass spectrometry for protein analysis. Methods Mol Biol 2006;328:131–9.

Salivary Biomarkers for the Detection of Malignant Tumors That are Remote from the Oral Cavity

Lenora R. Bigler, PhD, Charles F. Streckfus, DDS, MA*,
William P. Dubinsky, PhD

KEYWORDS

- Saliva • Breast cancer • Mass spectrometry • Diagnosis
- Biomarkers • Proteins • Cell signaling and pathways

Saliva is a complex and dynamic biologic fluid, which over the years has been recognized for the numerous functions it performs in the oral cavity. Modern technology, however, has unveiled a plethora of compounds never before detected in saliva (eg, drugs, pollutants, hormones; but also biomarkers of bacterial, viral, and systemic disease). Consequently, the increased scientific inquiry into salivary biomarkers has led to a more intense analysis of how saliva is collected, stored, and assayed and increased its potential use as a diagnostic medium in cancer research.[1]

In a recent review of the use of saliva as research material, Schipper and colleagues[2] discussed how over the past 50 years, the pace of salivary research has accelerated with the advent of new techniques that illuminate the biochemical and physicochemical properties of saliva. The field of salivary research is rapidly advancing because of the use of novel approaches that include metabolics, genomics, proteomics, and bioinformatics.

BLOOD VERSUS SALIVA AS A DIAGNOSTIC MEDIA

Blood has traditionally been the media of choice for the medical community and has, as a diagnostic media, served physicians very well over the decades. There may be some inherent disadvantages with blood, however, in biomarker discovery. Blood is basically in a closed loop (ie, the cardiovascular system), which contains numerous cells coursing through various organs that potentially can alter proteins that can exist within the circuit for a period of days or weeks. In comparison, the saliva is a

Department of Diagnostic Sciences, University of Texas Dental Branch at Houston, 6516 M.D. Anderson Boulevard, Room 4.133f, Houston, TX 77030, USA
* Corresponding author.
E-mail address: charles.streckfus@uth.tmc.edu (C.F. Streckfus).

Clin Lab Med 29 (2009) 71–85
doi:10.1016/j.cll.2009.01.004
0272-2712/09/$ – see front matter © 2009 Elsevier Inc. All rights reserved.

"real-time" fluid. The salivary glands are exocrine glands that produce protein profiles indicative of the individual's status at the moment of collection. This potentially may be an advantage when seeking biomarkers for various diseases.

ANALYTICAL ADVANTAGES OF SALIVA

Saliva as a diagnostic fluid has significant biochemical and logistical advantages when compared with blood. Biochemically, saliva is a clear liquid with an average protein concentration of 1.5 to 2 mg/mL. As a consequence of this low protein concentration, it was once assumed that this was a major drawback for using saliva as a diagnostic fluid; however, current ultrasensitive analyte detection techniques have eliminated this barrier. Saliva specimen preparation is simple, involving centrifugation before storage and the addition of a cocktail of protease inhibitors to reduce protein degradation for long-term storage.[3]

Blood is a far more complex medium. A decision has to be made as to whether to use serum or plasma. Serum has a total protein concentration of approximately 60 to 80 mg/mL. Because serum possesses more proteins than saliva, assaying trace amounts of factors (eg, oncogenes) may result in a greater risk of nonspecific interference and a greater chance for hydrostatic (and other) interactions between the factors and the abundant serum proteins. Serum also possesses numerous carrier proteins (eg, albumin), which must either be removed or treated before being assayed for protein content. Additionally, it was demonstrated that clotting removes many background proteins that may be altered in the presence of disease. It was established that enzymatic activity continues during this process, which may cleave many relevant pathway-related proteins.[4–6]

It would be ideal if all enzymatic activity in serum ceased at the time of collection; however, proteomic analyses of serum has shown that this is not the case. As a consequence, plasma is also being explored as a diagnostic fluid. The main consideration in using plasma is the selection of a proper anticoagulant.[4–6] Heparin, for example, can be used as an anticlotting agent; however, current research has found that heparin has a relatively short half-life (3–4 hours) and can produce products of coagulation that are abundantly comparable with those assayed in serum. Based on these observations, it is recommended that blood specimens be collected with ethylenediaminetetraacetic acid.

COLLECTION ADVANTAGES OF SALIVA

From a logistical perspective, the collection of saliva is safe (eg, no needle punctures), noninvasive, and relatively simple, and may be collected repeatedly without discomfort to the patient.[3] Consequently, it may be then possible to develop a simplified method for home-testing, testing in a health fair setting, or in dental clinics where individuals are available for periodic oral examinations. This diagnostic potential could reach many individuals who for personal, logistical, or economical reasons lack access to preventive care.[3]

Blood is more complicated to collect. It requires highly trained personnel to collect it and, if collected incorrectly, can lead to misinterpretations, which can result in patient mismanagement.[4–6] Blood specimens need to be collected in a specific sequence and under-filling tubes with additives; if not this may possibly alter protein analyses. Additionally, if specimens are collected during hospital or clinical settings, there may be a lapse of time from venipuncture to laboratory processing.[7]

PROTEOMIC ANALYSES OF SALIVA

From a biochemical point of view, proteins are the most important constituents of saliva. Currently, state-of-the art proteomic methods can be applied to the analysis of salivary peptides and proteins.

Recently, surface-enhanced laser desorption and ionization time-of-flight (SELDI-TOF) protein chips combines matrix-assisted laser desorption and ionization TOF mass spectrometry (MS) to surface chromatography.[1] This technology uses sample chips that display various kinds of chemically enriched and active surfaces that bind protein molecules based on established principles, such as ion exchange chromatography, metal ion affinity, and hydrophobic affinity. The technique enables rapid and high-throughput detection of critical proteins and peptides directly from crude mixtures without labor-intensive preprocessing. Furthermore, SELDI-TOF-MS is sensitive and requires only small amounts of sample compared with other proteomic techniques.[1,8,9]

Studies by Schipper and colleagues[8] have demonstrated that SELDI-TOF-MS could serve as an alternative, rapid, and high throughput proteomic approach to profile salivary proteins and peptides. Chips with anionic (CM10) treated surfaces were effective in binding salivary proteins in the range from 6000 to 16,000 m/z. The cationic (Q10) and hydrophobic (H4) chips were found to be most valuable for the characterization of saliva peptides and proteins in the low molecular (1000–6000 m/z) range. The metal affinity binding (IMAC-Cu) chip produced the highest number of peaks in a wide molecular range. SELDI technology enables selective protein retention on protein chip array surfaces by means of distinct chromatographic surfaces. Protein chip arrays are available with a variety of chromatographic surfaces including reverse phase, cation exchange, anion exchange, and immobilized metal affinity surfaces. Other arrays are available for covalent coupling of antibodies, DNA, RNA, receptors, or other "bait" molecules onto the array surface.[1,8,9]

Crude biologic samples can be applied directly to the protein chip arrays. After a short incubation period, unbound proteins are washed off the surface of the array. Only proteins that interact with the array chemical surface are retained for further analysis. Protein chip arrays are analyzed in the protein chip reader. The process involves laser desorption and ionization of proteins from the array surface, and detection by TOF-MS. The protein chip reader is a laser desorption and ionization TOF mass spectrometer that uses state-of-the-art ion optic and laser optic technology. The laser optics maximize ion extraction efficiency over the greatest possible sample area, and increase analytical sensitivity and reproducibility.[1,8,9]

The reader's ion optics incorporate a four-stage, time-lag focusing ion lens assembly that provides precise, accurate molecular weight determination with excellent mass sensitivity. Protein chip systems produce data compatible with all major protein databases and for applications requiring high sensitivity. Proteins can be quantified by plotting peak intensity values against peptide or protein standard quantities. The operating mechanism of ionic exchange protein chip arrays is the reversible binding of charged molecules to the surface, and the property of a peptide-protein that governs its binding is its net surface charge.[1,8,9] Because surface charge is the result of weak acidic and basic amino acids within the protein, binding of the protein to the array is highly pH dependent. Streckfus and colleagues[9] performed an analysis of a large number of saliva samples from women with and without breast cancer, which identified five mass peaks that were increased more than twofold in the cancer patients.

More recently, this same group has performed MS studies using saliva,[10,11] which when combined with previous work, corroborates earlier findings regarding the use of saliva as a medium for biomarkers of cancer.[12] In addition, two-dimensional gel electrophoresis and two-dimensional liquid chromatography (LC) coupled with tryptic digest analysis by MS have been demonstrated to be powerful proteomic tools for the global analysis of salivary proteins. The wide range of the molecular weights of salivary proteins necessitates additional methodologies, however (eg, high performance liquid chromatography [HPLC]-MS), particularly in the analysis of small proteins. The analysis is performed on an Applied Biosystems (Foster City, California) QStar XL LC tandem MS mass spectrometer equipped with an LC packings HPLC for capillary chromatography. The HPLC is coupled to the mass spectrometer by a nanospray electrospray ionization (ESI) head for maximal sensitivity.[13–15] The advantage of tandem MS combined with LC is enhanced sensitivity and the peptide separations afforded by chromatography. Even in complex protein mixtures, tandem MS data can be used to sequence and identify peptides either by peptide similarity or sequence analysis with a high degree of confidence.[13–17] This technique, albeit not a high-throughput technique, is far superior to the SELDI approach. The SELDI is challenged because of its small laser and has difficulty in spectral repeatability.

Several studies by Hu and colleagues[18] have used two-dimensional gel electrophoresis to separate the protein components followed by MS subsequently to identify the peptides produced from in-gel digests of the proteins of interest (two-dimensional MS). With this approach more than 300 proteins were identified in whole saliva. Although two-dimensional MS is a very powerful approach to protein separation, it has limitations when dealing with small-molecular-weight proteins, highly acidic or basic proteins, very hydrophobic proteins, or proteins in low abundance. In addition, the technique requires a relatively large amount of sample, is labor-intensive, and high gel-to-gel reproducibility is hard to achieve.

An alternative approach is the combination of LC as the separation step, with the mass spectrometer (LC-MS). Using this approach, more than 1000 peptides and proteins were identified including most known salivary proteins and serum proteins. This technique has the disadvantage that it is still labor intensive, has limited throughput, and provides little information about the relative abundance of the detected proteins. The initial salivary proteome profile of Hu and colleagues[19] was greatly expanded by combining LC-MS and two-dimensional MS, identifying more than 1050 proteins in whole saliva. LC methods coupled to MS or tandem MS are particularly suitable for separation and identification of low-molecular-weight components and peptides. These methods have allowed the detection of peptides in the range of 1 to 6 kd, many of which have important biologic functions (eg, histatins, cystatins, defensins, statherins, proline-rich proteins).

Along these lines, a consortium of three research groups lead by Denny and colleagues[20] cataloged the proteins in human saliva collected as the ductal secretions: 1166 identifications, 914 in parotid and 917 in submandibular-sublingual saliva, were made. The results showed that a high proportion of proteins that are found in plasma or tears are also present in saliva along with unique components. The proteins identified are involved in numerous molecular processes ranging from structural functions to enzymatic-catalytic activities. As expected, most mapped to the extracellular and secretory compartments. An immunoblot approach was used to validate the presence in saliva of a subset of the proteins identified by MS approaches. These experiments focused on novel constituents and proteins for which the peptide evidence was relatively weak.

Ultimately, information derived from the work reported here and related published studies can be used to translate blood-based clinical laboratory tests into a format that uses saliva. Additionally, a catalog of the salivary proteome of healthy individuals allows future analyses of salivary samples from individuals with oral and systemic diseases, with the goal of identifying biomarkers with diagnostic or prognostic value for these conditions; another possibility is the discovery of therapeutic targets.

The main goal to search for the complete protein salivary profile is its use as a diagnostic tool to monitor the physiologic, health, or disease status of individuals. With the advent of protein microarrays, spectra from a significant number of samples can be obtained and compared in a relatively short time with very little sample preparation or sophisticated chromatography.

Along these lines, cancer proteomics encompasses the identification and quantitative analysis of biomarkers, which are subsequently objectively measured indicators that characterize the state of health of the biologic system being analyzed. Because over 95% of all drug targets for varying carcinomas are proteins, the major goal of biomarker discovery or protein profiling is to identify disease-specific proteins and peptides from the proteome of biologic samples. Research has primarily focused on lower-molecular-weight proteins circulating within easily extractable body fluids, such as blood, urine, sputum, and saliva. The discovery of breast cancer markers in saliva has offered renewed interest in the potential use of saliva as a diagnostic fluid.

ISOTOPIC LABELING AND LIQUID CHROMATOGRAPHY TANDEM MASS SPECTROSCOPY

Isotopic labeling of protein mixtures has proved to be a useful technique for the analysis of relative expression levels of proteins in complex protein mixtures, such as saliva. There are two methods that are based on isotopically labeled protein modifying reagents to label or tag proteins in the mixtures: the iCAT and the iTRAQ techniques.[13–17]

The general approach for both techniques is to label two to four different saliva samples with agents that are chemically identical, but have different atomic masses. Any chemically based purification technique does not distinguish between the two; however, in the mass spectrometer they can be distinguished by their difference in atomic mass. Because they are chemically identical, they ionize with the same efficiency in the mass spectrometer permitting an estimate of their relative concentrations based on the relative peak intensities. iCAT procedure uses cysteine-specific labels that include a biotin moiety in their structure. An avidan binding step enables a high degree of enrichment of iCAT-labeled peptides.

The alternative to the iCAT procedure is the iTRAQ reagents, which are amino reactive compounds.[11,13–17] The real advantage is that the tag remains intact through TOF MS analysis; in the tandem MS spectrum for each peptide there is a fingerprint indicating the amount of that peptide from each of the different protein pools. Because virtually all of the peptides in a mixture are labeled by the reaction, numerous proteins in complex mixtures are identified and can be compared for their relative concentrations in each mixture; in these complex mixtures there is a high degree of confidence in the identification because of the large number of peptides that can be used for protein identification.[11,15–19]

The authors used IL-LC tandem MS technique to protein profile saliva for novel cancer-related biomarkers.[11,19] To identify potential salivary protein markers for the detection of breast cancer the following were used: pooled (N = 10) saliva specimens from healthy subjects; pooled (N = 10) saliva specimens from benign tumor patients (fibroadenomas); pooled (N = 10) saliva specimens from stage 0 cancer subjects; and pooled (N = 10) saliva specimens from stage I breast cancer subjects. An internal standard was created by pooling 10 specimens randomly selected from the pooled population. The analytical matrix is shown in **Fig. 1.**

iTRAQ Work Flow Schematic

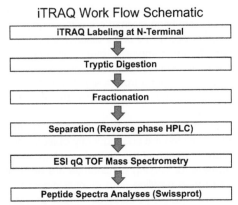

| iTRAQ Labeling at N-Terminal |
| Tryptic Digestion |
| Fractionation |
| Separation (Reverse phase HPLC) |
| ESI qQ TOF Mass Spectrometry |
| Peptide Spectra Analyses (Swissprot) |

Fig. 1. Steps for the iTRAQ proteomic procedure. ESI, electrospray ionization; HPLC, high performance liquid chromatography; TOF, time of flight.

The saliva samples were thawed and immediately centrifuged to remove insoluble materials. The supernatant was assayed for protein (Bio-Rad, San Diego, California) and an aliquot containing 100 µg of each specimen was precipitated with six volumes of −20°C acetone.

The precipitate was resuspended and treated according to the manufacturer's instructions. The treatment included blocking cysteine residues with methylmethane thiosulphate (MMTS) and trypsin digestion (**Fig. 2**). The peptides generated during the digestion were labeled with specifically coded iTRAQ reagents. The labeled peptides from each of the saliva samples were then combined and partially purified by a combination of cation exchange chromatography and desalting on a reverse phase column. The desalted and concentrated peptide mixtures were analyzed by MS.

Before MS an aliquot of the peptide mixture was separated by HPLC on a C18 75-µ × 10-cm reverse phase capillary column (Vydac 218MS3.07510). A linear gradient of 2% to 50% acetonitrile in 0.1% formic acid, over 180 minutes followed by 40 minutes

Analytical Strategy

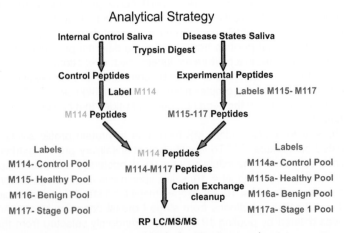

Fig. 2. Analytical comparisons associated with the iTRAQ procedure.

wash with 2% acetonitrile was used to elute the peptides directly into the mass spectrometer for tandem MS analysis. The QSTAR operates in an information-dependent acquisition mode, which detects peptides by TOF-MS and then fragments them by collision-induced dissociation in the tandem MS mode. The accumulated tandem MS spectra were analyzed by ProQuant (Applied Biosystems).

Table 1 shows the results of the experiment using pooled saliva samples. Overall 70 proteins were identified at greater than 99% confidence level (two or more peptides sequenced at >99% confidence interval) and 209 proteins at greater than 95% confidence level (at least one peptide sequenced at >99% confidence interval). These findings are slightly higher than Wilmarth and coworkers'[13] findings using a two-dimensional LC technique with LC tandem MS.

The internal standards and their resultant protein profiles were compared and produced similar results. Likewise, the healthy and benign subject spectra between the two runs were also comparable demonstrating reliable and reproducible data for additional spectral comparisons across the two individual runs. As illustrated in **Table 2**, the healthy subjects were labeled with a 115 marker, the benign subjects with a 116 marker, and the cancer groups with the 117 marker. Comparisons are listed in **Table 2**. A list of candidate up- and down-regulated proteins is listed in **Tables 3** and **4**.

The proteins were entered into Ingenuity software, pathway analysis software application that enables researchers to model, analyze, and understand the complex biologic and chemical systems at the core of cancer research. The results of the analyses are in **Figs. 3** and **4**. **Fig. 3** shows an association with the epidermal growth factor (epidermal growth factor [EGF]) pathway, which is at the heart of carcinogenesis, whereas **Fig. 4** suggests associations with the ubiquitin pathway. As illustrated, the proteins are associated with varying pathways that are common to both the ductal epithelia of the breast and the ductal epithelia of the salivary glands. Additionally, these same proteins have been found to be either up- or down-regulated in MCF-7 and SKBR-3 cancer cell lines. Interestingly, results identified proteins that are both up- or down-regulated, have varying cellular functions, and have been validated in cell studies to be altered in the presence of carcinoma of the breast.[11]

THE SALIVARY GLAND MODEL

The ideas outlined previously lead to the question as to what the possible mechanisms of action are in relation to models involving salivary diagnostics and breast cancer development. First, one should examine the similarities that salivary and breast tissue, and fluids from each, have in common. Pia-Foshini and colleagues[21] describe how breast glands and salivary glands are both tubuloacinar exocrine glands sharing similar morphologic features; consequently, it is reasonable to expect similarities in pathologic processes. They differ in incidence and clinical behavior, however,

Table 1					
Liquid chromatography mass spectrometry/mass spectrometry experiment results					
Confidence	Proteins	Before Grouping	Peptides	Spectra	% Total Spectra
>99	70	966	478	1099	73.6
>95	209	1674	626	1329	89
>66	351	1978	772	1491	99.9
As shown: >95	209	1674	626	1329	89

Table 2
Comparison of healthy subjects, benign subjects, and cancer groups

Comparison	Up-Regulated	Down-Regulated	Total Markers
Healthy versus benign	19	10	29
Healthy versus stage 0	15	15	30
Healthy versus stage I	9	17	26
Benign versus cancers	9	6	15

depending on whether they are primary in breast or the salivary glands. Salivary gland–like tumors of the breast are of two types: myoepithelial differentiation and those devoid of myoepithelial differentiation. Myoepithelial differentiated tumors comprise a spectrum of lesions from pleomorphic adenoma to low-grade adenosquamous carcinoma, whereas nonmyoepithelial differentiated tumors are rare acinic cell carcinomas. Nicol and Iskandar[22] describe lobular carcinoma of the breast metastatic to the oral cavity mimicking polymorphous low-grade adenocarcinoma of the minor salivary glands.

Table 3
Candidate up and down proteins

Accession	Protein Name	Ratio	P Value
Q9DCT1	Aldo-keto reductase	1.3874	0.0264
P04083	Annexin A1	3.0606	0.0001
P23280	Carbonic anhydrase VI	1.5160	0.0003
P01040	Cystatin A	2.0057	0.0014
P01036	Cystatin SA-III	1.2030	0.0115
Q7NXI3	Heat shock 70kDa protein	1.2732	0.0039
Q01469	Epidermal fatty acid-binding protein	2.0963	0.0362
Q6LAF3	Histone H4	2.4094	0.0059
P01857	Ig gamma-1 chain C region	1.4396	0.0034
P13646	Cytokeratin 13	6.5643	0.0001
P19013	Cytokeratin 4	6.4958	0.0019
P48666	Cytokeratin 6C	4.4113	0.0001
P01871	Ig mu chain C region	1.5134	0.0011
Q9HC84	Mucin 5B	1.6771	0.0001
P05164	Myeloperoxidase precursor	2.7188	0.0005
P31151	S100 calcium-binding protein	2.0519	0.0001
P05109	Calgranulin A	2.1848	0.0001
P06702	Calgranulin B	1.8686	0.0001
Q9UBC9	Cornifin beta	1.8252	0.0001
P02788	Lactoferrin	1.5766	0.0001
P00760	Cationic trypsin precursor	1.1572	0.0144
P68197	Ubiquitin	1.5533	0.0138

Table 4
Candidate up and down proteins

Accession	Protein Name	Ratio	P Value
P10981	Actin-87E	0.7657	0.0107
Q8N4F0	Bactericidal/permeability-increasing protein-like 1	0.7953	0.0004
Q9GQM9	Cytochrome P450	0.7277	0.0001
P04264	Cytokeratin 1	0.6106	0.0001
P01034	Cystatin C	0.7201	0.0187
P28325	Cystatin D precursor	0.6856	0.0010
Q71SP7	Fatty acid synthase	0.0311	0.0500
P00738	Haptoglobin	0.8266	0.0023
P22079	Lactoperoxidase	0.8247	0.0388
Q96DR5	Lipocalin	0.6144	0.0001
P79180	Lysozyme C	0.5309	0.0031
P07737	Profilin-1	0.6752	0.0135
P02768	Serum albumin precursor	0.7336	0.0001
P02787	Transferrin	0.7192	0.0001
P25311	Zinc-alpha-2-glycoprotein	0.8454	0.0009

Furthermore, Bretschneider and colleagues[23] report studies that suggest breast cancer and salivary gland tumors share an expression pattern unique to these two tissues (eg, BASE and SBEM). BASE encodes a putative secreted protein that is restricted to breast cancer cells and salivary gland. It seems to be estrogen receptor alpha dependent in its expression and may offer clues to how multiple disease states at distant locations can share similar mechanisms of expression and regulation.

With these studies in mind, Miksicek and colleagues[24] suggest that improving the diagnosis and clinical management of breast cancer requires access to a wider range of biomarkers able to reflect the molecular phenotype of breast tissue. A special mRNA identified only in mammary and salivary glands is termed "small breast epithelial mucin." Secreted proteins that contain internally repeated densely glycosylated neutral core motifs have a well-established link to cancer as illustrated by the MUC1 gene product. This study identifies a novel breast and salivary gland–specific, mucin-like gene that is strongly expressed in normal and tumor human mammary epithelium. Furthermore, Amundadottir and colleagues[25] report a basic science study using transgenics that demonstrates cooperation between oncogenic proteins c-*myc* and transforming growth factor-α in mouse mammary and salivary gland tumorigenesis. The protein product of c-*myc* is responsible for transcriptional activation of cells and transforming growth factor-α is part of the EGF family and activates the EGF receptor, whose overexpression is associated with poor prognosis and high degree of invasiveness in breast cancer.

Noble and colleagues[26] published a pilot study that examined the feasibility of nipple aspiration to distinguish women with breast cancer from healthy women using surface-enhanced laser desorption ionization TOF-MS. Nipple aspiration fluid was collected from each breast in 21 women newly diagnosed with unilateral breast cancer and 44 healthy women. No differences were found when proteomic profiles of nipple aspiration fluid from the cancer-bearing breast and the contralateral noncancerous

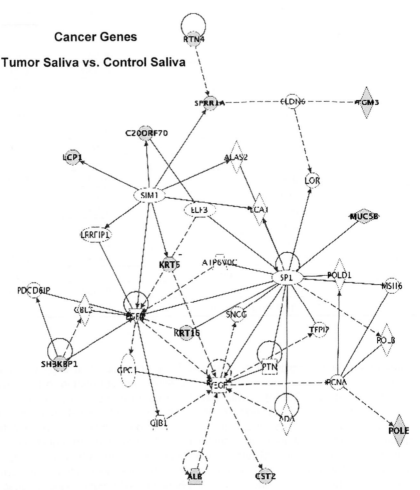

Fig. 3. Up-regulated growth pathways associated with the salivary protein profile in the presence of carcinoma of the breast.

breast were compared. In contrast, nine protein peaks were significantly different between the cancer-bearing breast compared with healthy women and 10 peaks were significantly different between the contralateral healthy breast and healthy women (P<.05). These data suggest that invasive breast cancer may result in a field change across both breasts and that proteomic profiling of nipple aspiration fluid may have more value in breast cancer risk assessment than as a diagnostic or screening tool.

In addition, Medrinos and colleagues[27] described a study that focused on an innovative technique that couples breast ductal lavage with surface-enhanced laser desorption and ionization TOF-MS to yield a highly sensitive and specific method of breast carcinoma detection. The study group included 16 women who had unilateral, biopsy-proved breast carcinoma. Studying paired ductal lavage specimens from each woman (the breast with and the breast without carcinoma); a cytologic investigation was performed on the cells present in the ductal lavage samples; and the protein content of the ductal lavage fluid was analyzed with the SELDI-TOF-MS technique

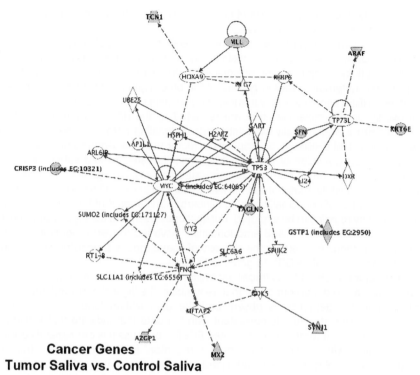

Cancer Genes
Tumor Saliva vs. Control Saliva

Fig. 4. Down-regulated apoptotic pathways associated with the salivary protein profile in the presence of carcinoma of the breast.

using the strong anionic exchange chip surface. Only five (31%) of 16 ductal lavage specimens from breasts with biopsy-proved carcinoma contained malignant cells, whereas the remaining samples contained only histiocytes and clusters of benign ductal epithelium. In contrast, 12 (75%) of 16 ductal lavage specimens from breasts that contained carcinoma had a different protein peak pattern compared with the paired ductal lavage specimen from the same patient's contralateral, uninvolved breast. This finding was independent of the presence of neoplastic cells in the lavage fluid. In addition, specific protein peaks, which may represent potential biomarkers, were identified in the ductal lavage fluids from breasts with carcinoma. Some of these peaks were conserved between different patients. The study suggests cross-talk from the diseased breast to the healthy breast, which also produced an altered nipple aspiration fluid protein profile.

Finally, there are several hypothetical mechanisms that may explain the presence of novel biomarkers in saliva. Because there are numerous putative salivary proteins that are possibly altered in the presence of disease, the authors focus the discussion on salivary EGF, EGFR, and HER-2/neu because these proteins have been investigated and are molecularly associated with one another.[1]

EGFR (erbB-1) and HER-2/neu (erbB-2) are members of the ErbB tyrosine kinase receptor family comprising four related receptors (erbB-1, erbB-2, erbB-3, erbB-4). Collectively, they dimerize on ligand stimulation (EGF) and transduce their signals by subsequent autophosphorylation that catalyzes the receptor cytoplasmic tyrosine kinase activity, which results in the recruitment of an array of downstream signaling cascades. The type and amplitude of activated downstream activity is related to the type of receptor expressed by a cell.

Hynes and Lane[28] report that none of the EGF family of peptides bind ERBB2; however, MUC4, a member of the mucin family, acts as an intramembrane modulator of ERBB2 activity. Despite having no soluble ligand, ERBB2 is important because it is the preferred heterodimerization partner of the other ligand-bound family members. Activated ERBBs stimulate many intracellular signaling pathways and, despite extensive overlap in the molecules that are recruited to the different active receptors, different ERBBs preferentially modulate certain signaling pathways, because of the ability of individual ERBBs to bind specific effector proteins. Amplification of *ERBB2* leading to overexpression of the receptor, originally detected in a subset of breast tumors, occurs in other human cancers, such as ovarian, gastric, and salivary cancers.[28] Intriguingly, mutations in the kinase domain of *ERBB2* have been identified in a small number of non–small cell lung cancers.[28] The impact of these mutations on ERBB2 activity remains to be explored. Publications describing the crystal structure of the EGFR, ERBB2, and ERBB3 ectodomains[28] have led to new insights into some intriguing questions concerning the process of ligand-induced receptor dimerization and biologic activity of ERBB2-targeted antibodies.

The structure of ERBB2's extracellular region is radically different from the others. ERBB2 has a fixed conformation that resembles the ligand-activated state: the domain II to IV interaction is absent and the dimerization loop in domain II is exposed.[28,29] This structure is consistent with the data that indicate that ERBB2 is the preferred partner for the other activated ERBBs, because it is permanently poised for interaction with another ligand-bound receptor. Furthermore, this structure explains why no soluble EGF-related ligand has been found. It predicts that ERBB2 possesses a unique subdomain I to III interaction that makes ligand binding impossible because the site is buried and not accessible for interaction. To date, although HER-2/*neu* does not have a specific, known ligand, EGF, transforming growth factor-α, and the neuregulins are afew of the ligands that activate the erbB-1, erbB-3, and erbB-4 receptors. These receptors are present on both the ductal epithelium of breast and the ductal epithelium of the salivary glands and in the case of EGFR and HER-2/*neu* they can both be overexpressed in the presence of carcinoma respective to their tissues. The receptors can also be identified by using immunohistochemistry and have been clearly shown on both types of tissues. Along these lines, Hynes and Lane[28] and Lee-Hoeflich and colleagues[29] examined the central role for HER3 in HER2-amplified breast cancer with regard to targeted therapy regimens. They report using receptor knockdown by a small interfering RNA technology in cell lines to demonstrate that EGFR and HER3 each form heterodimers with HER2 and that inhibition of HER2 expression could be achieved by dual HER2/EGFR small molecule inhibitors.

It should be noted that breast cancer is not the only malignancy involving HER2 expression. Wang and colleagues[30] used tissue microarrays and immunohistochemical analysis to study protein expression of genes in the erb-b signaling pathway (erb-b1; erb-b2; phosphoinositide-3-kinase, catalytic, α polypeptide [PIK3CA]; phosphatase and tensin homolog [PTEN]; phosphorylated AKT [p-AKT]; and phosphorylated extracellular signal-regulated kinase [p-ERK]) in 118 advanced ovarian carcinomas and related expression to clinicopathologic features and survival. High protein expression was seen in 15.3% of cases for erb-b2, 44.1% for erb-b1, 43.2% for PIK3CA, 51.6% for p-AKT, and 28% for p-ERK. Low protein levels of PTEN were seen in 41.5% of the cases and tended to be more common in well-differentiated tumors. In multivariate analysis, only high expression of both erb-b1 and erb-b2 was an independent factor in progression-free and disease-specific survival (P = .009, hazard ratio = 2.46; P = .002, hazard ratio = 3.023, respectively). The PI3 K/AKT and RAS/MEK/ERK pathways seem to be activated in some cases of advanced ovarian carcinomas, although PIK3CA, p-AKT, p-ERK, and PTEN do not seem to be independent prognostic markers in this group of patients. By using tissue microarrays and immunohistochemical assessment, high expression of both erb-b1 and erb-b2 was an independent prognostic factor in advanced ovarian carcinomas. High activation of PI3 K/AKT and RAS/MEK/ERK pathways was detected in advanced ovarian carcinomas. PIK3CA, p-AKT, p-ERK, and PTEN did not seem to be independent prognostic markers, however, in this group of patients.

Using EGF, EGFR, and HER-2/*neu* as a molecular model, the authors postulate that in the presence of disease (eg, carcinoma of the breast) there is an overabundance of protein resulting from the rapid growth of the malignancy, which in turn produces a humoral response in the salivary glands. This response results in altered salivary protein concentrations. Another possible explanation is active transport of the proteins of interest. It is plausible that these proteins are secreted into saliva as consequence of localized regulatory function in the oral cavity by signal transduction similar to the proposed explanation of HER-2/*neu* protein in nipple aspirates. These "loop" mechanisms, in health, seem to be in equilibrium both intercellularly and extracellularly with each pathway fulfilling the resultant phenotypic process of growth, proliferation, and differentiation.

Yet another possible mechanism of action is passive diffusion of proteins from the serum to the saliva across the cell membranes. Considering the general molecular size of the aforementioned proteins, it is very unlikely proteins of their magnitude would passively diffuse into salivary secretions.

This leaves active transport of proteins from serum to saliva and whether HER-2/*neu* in saliva could have used a similar mechanism as endosomal sorting complex required for transport is an intriguing possibility. Trajkovic and coworkers[31] established a pathway in intraendosomal membrane transport and exosome formation that required the sphingolipid ceramide. Lysosomal degradation of proteins following endocytosis is preceded by the incorporation of the proteins into intraluminal vesicles of multivesicular endosomes and delivered to lysosomes for digestion. Alternatively, the multivesicular endosomes can directly fuse with the plasma membrane, releasing the intraluminal vesicles to the extracellular environment as exosomes and thereby functioning as intercellular signaling. These studies indicate that proteolipid protein-containing exosomes and epidermal growth factor receptor–containing intraluminal vesicles can be formed within the same endosome.[31] Salivary HER2 and other oncogenic proteins could feasibly use a similar route, but no studies have been conducted to date. Currently, relatively little is known about the signals and mechanisms that initiate protein secretion of these nonoral related proteins. Until these and other questions are answered, one can only postulate as to how and why these large proteins are secreted into the oral cavity.

REFERENCES

1. Streckfus CF, Bigler L. The use of soluble, salivary c-erbB-2 for the detection and post-operative follow-up of breast cancer in women: the results of a five year translational study. Adv Dent Res 2005;18:17–22.
2. Schipper R, Silletti E, Vingerhoeds MH. Saliva as research material: biochemical, physicochemical and practical aspects. Arch Oral Biol 2007;52:1114–35.
3. Streckfus CF, Bigler L. Saliva as a diagnostic fluid. Oral Dis 2002;8(2):69–76.

4. Koomen JM, Li D, Xiao L, et al. Direct tandem mass spectrometry reveals limitations in protein profiling experiments for plasma biomarker recovery. J Proteome Res 2005;4(3):972–81.

5. Teisner B, Davey MW, Grudzinskas JG. Interaction between heparin and plasma proteins analyzed by crossed immunoelectrophoresis and affinity chromatography. Clin Chim Acta 1983;127(3):413–7.

6. Srinivas PR, Srivastava S, Hanash S, et al. Proteomics in early detection of cancer. Clin Chem 2001;47(10):1901–11.

7. Ernst DJ, Balance LO. Quality collection: the phlebotomist's role in pre-analytical errors. MLO Med Lab Obs 2006;83(9):30–8.

8. Schipper R, Loof A, De Groot J, et al. SELDI-TOF-MS of saliva: methodology and pre-treatment effects. J Chromatogr B Analyt Technol Biomed Life Sci 2007;847: 46–53.

9. Streckfus CF, Bigler LR, Zwick M. The use of surface enhanced laser desorption/ ionization time-of-flight mass spectrometry to detect putative breast cancer markers in saliva: a feasibility study. J Oral Pathol Med 2006;35:292–300.

10. Streckfus CF, Dubinsky W. Proteomic analysis of saliva for cancer diagnosis. Expert Rev Proteomics 2007;4(3):329–32.

11. Streckfus CF, Mayorga-Wark O, Daniel Arreola D, et al. Breast cancer related proteins are present in saliva and are modulated secondary to ductal carcinoma in situ of the breast. Cancer Invest 2008;26(2):159–67.

12. Streckfus CF, Bigler L, Dellinger TD, et al. The presence of c-erbB-2, and CA 15–3 in saliva and serum among women with breast carcinoma: a preliminary study. Clin Cancer Res 2000;6(6):2363–70.

13. Wilmarth PA, Riviere MA, Rustvold DL, et al. Two dimensional liquid chromatography study of the human whole saliva proteome. J Proteome Res 2004;3:1017–23.

14. Gu S, Liu Z, Pan S, et al. Global investigation of p53-induced apoptosis through quantitative proteomic profiling using comparative amino acid-coded tagging. Mol Cell Proteomics 2004;10:998–1008.

15. Shevchenko A, Chernushevic I, Shevchenko A, et al. De novo sequencing of peptides recovered from in-gel digested proteins by nanoelectrospray tandem mass spectrometry. Mol Biotechnol 2002;20:107–18.

16. Koomen JM, Zhao H, Li D, et al. Diagnostic protein discovery using proteolytic peptide targeting and identification. Rapid Commun Mass Spectrom 2004;18: 2537–48.

17. Ward LD, Reid GE, Moritz RL, et al. Strategies for internal amino acid sequence analysis of proteins separated by polyacrylamide gel electrophoresis. J Chromatogr 1990;519:199–216.

18. Hu S, Li Y, Wong DT, et al. Large-scale identification of proteins in human salivary proteome by liquid chromatography/mass spectrometry and two-dimensional gel electrophoresis-mass spectrometry. Proteomics 2005;5:1714–28.

19. Hu S, Loo JA, Wong DT. Human saliva proteome analysis. Ann N Y Acad Sci 2007;1098:323–9.

20. Denny P, Hagen FK, Hardt M, et al. The proteomes of human parotid and submandibular/sublingual gland salivas collected as the ductal secretions. J Proteome Res 2008;7(5):1994–2006.

21. Pia-Foschini M, Reis-Filho JS, Eusebi V, et al. Salivary gland-like tumours of the breast: surgical and molecular pathology. J Clin Pathol 2003;56:497–506.

22. Nicol KK, Iskandar SS. Lobular carcinoma of the breast metastatic to the oral cavity mimicking polymorphous low-grade adenocarcinoma of the minor salivary glands. Arch Pathol Lab Med 2000;124:157–9.

23. Bretschneider N, Brand H, Miller N, et al. Estrogen induces repression of the breast cancer and salivary gland expression gene in an estrogen receptor a-dependent manner. Cancer Res 2008;68(1):106–14.
24. Miksicek RJ, Myal Y, Watson PH, et al. Identification of a novel breast-and salivary gland-specific, mucin-like gene strongly expressed in normal and tumor human mammary epithelium. Cancer Res 2002;62:2736–40.
25. Amundadottir LR, Johnson MD, Merlino G, et al. Synergistic interaction of transforming growth factor a and c-myc in mouse mammary and salivary gland tumorigenesis. Cell Growth Differ 1995;6:737–48.
26. Noble JL, Dua RS, Coulton GR, et al. A comparative proteinomic analysis of nipple aspiration fluid from healthy women and women with breast cancer. Eur J Cancer 2007;43(16):2315–20.
27. Mendrinos S, Nolen JD, Styblo T, et al. Cytologic findings and protein expression profiles associated with ductal carcinoma of the breast in ductal lavage specimens using surface-enhanced laser desorption and ionization-time of flight mass spectrometry. Cancer 2005;105(3):178–83.
28. Hynes N, Lane H. ERBB receptors and cancer: the complexity of targeted inhibitors. Nat Rev Cancer 2005;5(5):341–54.
29. Lee-Hoeflich ST, Crocker L, Yao E, et al. A central role for HER3 in HER2-amplified breast cancer: implications for targeted therapy. Cancer Res 2008;68:5878–87.
30. Wang Y, Kristensen GB, Helland A, et al. Protein expression and prognostic value of genes in the erb-b signaling pathway in advanced ovarian carcinomas. Am J Clin Pathol 2005;124(3):392–401.
31. Trajkovic K, Hsu C, Chiantia S, et al. Ceramide triggers budding of exosome vesicles into multivesicular endosomes. Science 2008;319:1244–7.

Cardiovascular Proteomics: Implications for Clinical Applications

Florian S. Schoenhoff, MD[a,b], Qin Fu, PhD[a], Jennifer E. Van Eyk, PhD[a],*

KEYWORDS

- Proteomics • Biomarkers • Cardiac markers
- Multiplex assays • Discovery • Validation
- Translational research

Cardiovascular proteomics is a rapidly evolving field within life sciences. During the last decade, proteomics has been driven by the advent of new techniques in mass spectrometry (MS), and advances in classic techniques (eg, one- and two-dimensional protein separation gel electrophoresis and liquid chromatography).

Proteomics aims to identify and characterize the set of proteins present at a certain point in time. Unlike the mere identification of a gene, proteomics is extremely complex, requiring many technologies and strategies. Most genes, once they are expressed, undergo extensive posttranslational modification; this results in different functional gene products arising from the same gene. So far, there are 560 types of posttranslational modifications that can be detected by MS alone, with oxidation and phosphorylation being the most common ones. The number of possible protein variants from a single gene further increases when all splice variants are taken into account. A functional change is typically preceded by a change on the protein level, and this can be induced by the slightest fluctuation in the microenvironment of the protein (eg, change in pH). The strength of proteomics to detect these sometimes minute changes is at the same time the weakness of the method when translated to

---

Jennifer Van Eyk's work is supported by the National Heart Lung Blood Institute Proteomic Initiative (contract N01-HV-28,120), the SCCOR program (Specialized Centers of Clinically Oriented Research, grant 1 P50 HL 084,946-01), the Clinical Translational Science Award (#1U54RR023561-01A1) and by the Daniel P. Amos Foundation. Florian Schoenhoff is supported by the Novartis Research Foundation and the Swiss National Science Foundation (#PBSKP3-124604).

[a] The Johns Hopkins Bayview Proteomics Center, Division of Cardiology, Department of Medicine, Johns Hopkins University, 5200 Eastern Avenue, MFL Building, Suite 602, Baltimore, MD 21224, USA
[b] Department of Cardiovascular Surgery, University of Berne, Berne, Switzerland, Freiburgstrasse, 3010 Berne, Switzerland
* Corresponding author.
E-mail address: jvaneyk1@jhmi.edu (J.E. Van Eyk).

Clin Lab Med 29 (2009) 87–99
doi:10.1016/j.cll.2009.01.005
0272-2712/09/$ – see front matter © 2009 Elsevier Inc. All rights reserved.

the "real-world" context of a clinical setting. This article addresses the safeguards and pitfalls involved in taking proteomics from bench to bedside.

Most clinicians tend to underestimate the efforts that are necessary to conduct a proteomics study. Proteomics is often presented as a high-throughput single method, which (although it uses high-throughput techniques) it is not. The goal of proteomics is not speed but rather breadth of observation. Proteomics can simultaneously investigate tens, hundreds, even thousands of proteins. Because proteomics techniques are able to detect even the slightest changes in protein conformation (eg, posttranslational modifications), the methods themselves are sensitive to very slight modifications, and extreme care must be taken to achieve reproducible results. Over the last several years, plasma and serum have become the most common sample types for routine clinical use, because they are quite easy to obtain and provide a good reference for systemic processes.

One challenge with serum and plasma is the sheer depth of the proteome. The human genome project has identified only approximately 30,000 genes; but human plasma contains about 10^6 different molecules, and the concentrations of proteins in the plasma span nine magnitudes (from <1 pg/mL up to 50 mg/mL). Currently, there is no proteomics technique with a dynamic range that even comes close to covering these differences in protein abundance. Even after removing the 10 most abundant proteins (which account for 90% of the total protein content in the blood), analysis of the mid- and low-abundance proteins is feasible but challenging.[1] Although this makes proteomics seem, on first view, like a less-than-ideal candidate for clinical applications, this strategy has been incorporated into many biomarker studies based on the assumption that potentially interesting biomarkers are still hidden from standard proteomic techniques.

Biomarker discovery is conducted along two lines: one is the systems biology approach, driven by identifying all protein differences between disease and control; the other is a more targeted approach. Although several authors argue for one or the other, most researchers combine the two approaches.[2] The known biology of the disease informs choices as to the sample type, the collection method, and the proteomic techniques to be used. After the initial phase of discovery work, candidate markers are evaluated on the basis of the underlying biology, insofar as it is known. Proteins with pre-existing availability of antibodies and ELISA kits are often preferentially selected for validation. The need for highly specific antibodies presents a considerable and unfortunate bias in biomarker discovery, because this should not be the default selection criterion. Tools that can develop robust ELISAs in a timely fashion, and MS-based methods that allow for absolute quantification of proteins, are required. Indeed, there is considerable ongoing effort to overcome some of the difficulties in this area.

DE NOVO DISCOVERY

Biomarker discovery[3–6] uses one or more proteomics techniques to detect as many changes as possible between the proteomes of the disease and the control.[7,8] To achieve this, the essence of biomarker discovery methodology is to investigate two samples that differ only in one characteristic: the disease. Sample processing (**Fig. 1**) differs according to the nature of the sample (serum, plasma, cells, or tissue) and other case-specific factors, such as the biology of the disease.[9] In general, samples undergo analysis using a gel-based or gel-free approach either using protein or peptide methods.

In a gel-based approach, the proteins are separated in the first dimension by their isoelectric point, and then in the second dimension according to their mass within

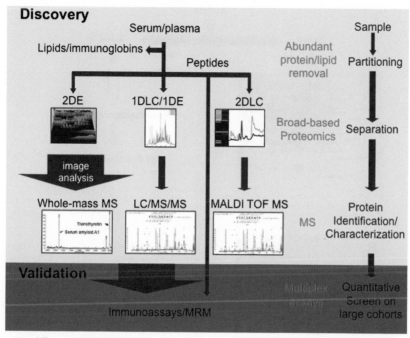

Fig. 1. Workflow in biomarker discovery and validation using proteomics techniques.

a polyacrylamide gel (SDS-PAGE). Today, most research groups use strips with fixed pH-gradients; these have been a tremendous improvement over ampholyte-based gradients, which are prone to instability over time. Fixed pH-gradient strips are available in several pH-ranges, so that a very high resolution can be achieved if the isoelectric point of the proteins in question is known in advance. At this point, the spots on the gel (each containing several proteins) represent all of the proteins in the sample. Depending on their intended use, the gels are now stained with silver, Coomassie blue, or more elaborate techniques like fluorescent dyes. Computer-assisted analysis of the gels identifies spots containing proteins of interest; these can then be excised, digested using trypsin, and subjected to further analysis by MS. Although there are limits to the dynamic range of the method, its ability to detect posttranslational modifications makes it worthwhile. A gel-free approach could accomplish separation of the sample's proteins by liquid chromatography coupled with tandem MS.

Once an individual combination of peptides is identified, the result is cross-referenced with protein databases to identify the protein in question. Because the overlap between gel-based and gel-free methods is only approximately 40%, combining protein separation methods enhances the breadth of protein coverage.

Regardless of the peptide or protein approach, and to enhance the depth of coverage in proteomes isolated from cells, samples are fractionated into subproteomes[10] by a process, such as enrichment of mitochondrial or myofilament fractions. Depletion of samples from the most abundant proteins can increase the resolution of the subsequent proteomics technique. Several protocols have been developed to deplete serum and plasma samples from albumin and immunoglobulins, by either chemical means (using sodium chloride and ethanol) or affinity-based methods (Fig. 2). Recent research on the "albuminome" raises questions about this methodology, however, showing that several important proteins are actually bound to albumin

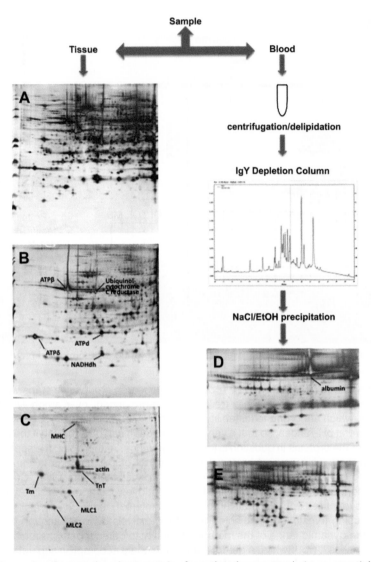

Fig. 2. Removing the top abundant proteins from the plasma sample is an essential step in enhancing sensitivity and depth of coverage of the downstream techniques. In tissue samples, this can be achieved by enriching the sample for certain subproteomes. (*A*) Silver-stained two-dimensional PAGE image of homogenized cardiac tissue. (*B*) Silver-stained two-dimensional PAGE image of mitochondria-enriched fractions. (*C*) Myofilament-enriched fractions in blue-silver staining (*Courtesy of* G. Agnetti, Johns Hopkins University, Baltimore, MD). (*D*) Two-dimensional PAGE image of albumin-associated retenate after depletion of human plasma. (*E*) The protein separation of the depleted plasma itself.

and are removed with it from the sample. Furthermore, the "albuminome" has been linked with cardiovascular disease, suggesting that investigation of albumin samples may be fruitful in and of itself.

The importance of preanalytical issues in proteomics is often underestimated; such issues play a major role in successful proteomics studies, especially when dealing with complex matrices, such as plasma or serum. The two keys to reducing preanalytical variation are consistency and thorough knowledge of the underlying biology. Samples must be harvested under precisely the same conditions, controlling for time point (circadian rhythm); pH; temperature; posture (supine versus upright); and equipment (eg, syringes, needles, and tubes). Processing must follow a similarly strict protocol. The purpose of the analysis, and the characteristics of the potential analytes, should be kept in mind when selecting the sample type. For example, serum is easy to obtain, but because of ex vivo processes (eg, formation of additional peptides, or binding of proteins to the blood clot) it might not be ideal for proteomics-based biomarker discovery; in such cases, plasma should be preferred.[11] The main anticoagulants used in the preparation of plasma are citrate, ethylenediaminetetraacetic acid, and heparin, but each of these additives limits the usability of the sample. Citrate binds Ca^{2+} and has been shown to interfere with immunoassays[12]; and ethylenediaminetetraacetic acid can preclude the analysis of such enzymes as matrix metalloproteinases, because the chelating properties inhibit the cofactors of the enzyme. In 2005, the HUPO Plasma Proteome Project published a comprehensive study[13] on sample protocols and varying experimental conditions. An overview of the preanalytical factors found to influence proteomics-based biomarker discovery is given in **Box 1**. As stated, the underlying biology (as exemplified by the variance in transforming growth factor-β levels when using polystyrene instead of polypropylene plates, because of the interaction of the protein with different surfaces) also plays a major role in analysis and technique.

For use in a clinical setting, it is very important to plan and implement a protocol that is feasible in the field, and yet yields scientifically meaningful results. **Box 2** depicts a protocol (for collecting samples for proteomics analysis) that has been successfully implemented in the cardiac surgery operating rooms of the authors' institution. Although there is no broad evidence regarding the optimal storage temperatures for proteomic samples, they strongly recommend storage at −80°C Because repeated freeze-thaw cycles have a detectable and deleterious effect on the protein content of the samples, appropriate aliquoting of the initial sample should be one of the first steps in consistent processing of samples. Access to liquid nitrogen and sophisticated, cooled centrifuges may constitute a particular problem in routine clinical workflows. Initial storage of the centrifuged sample at −80°C, followed by aliquoting and snap-freezing in liquid nitrogen in a laboratory environment, presents a compromise that requires only minimal time in the operating room while effectively preserving sample quality for further analysis. It should be noted that even approved, standard laboratory operating procedures (ie, National Committee for Clinical Laboratory Standards) are sometimes not sufficient for proteomics analysis. A popular example is the family of the transforming growth factors (transforming growth factor-β), which have recently received attention for their involvement in several key biologic processes.[14] Transforming growth factor-β is released ex vivo from platelets, and samples must be platelet-free to ensure that transforming growth factor-β levels are not overestimated. One could argue that if a biomarker is not robust enough to survive small deviations from a protocol, it is inherently not useful for the clinical routine. Although this might hold true for the strict validation part of a proteomics study, it seriously hampers any attempts at biomarker discovery using a proteomics approach.

VALIDATION AND VERIFICATION OR TARGETED DISCOVERY

After identification of candidate markers during the discovery stage, the proteins are forwarded to validation or verification. Validation is performed to confirm that protein identification is consistent with the way the protein is actually represented in the sample. Validation of MS-based protein identifications can be misleading, because

Box 1
Preanalytical factors influencing proteomics-based techniques

Patient information

- Gender
- Age
- Diet
- Genetics
- Medical background
- Health background
- Pregnancy, menopausal
- Medications
- Alcohol intake, smoking status
- Fasting, postprandial

Phlebotomy

- Tourniquest technique
- Seated, standing, lying
- Tube order: first versus last
- Drawn from existing line

Collective device

- Glass or plastic tube
- Gel or nongel separator
- Tube additives

Blood derivative and processing

- Plasma versus serum
- Ethylenediaminetetraacetic acid versus citrate versus heparin
- Clotting procedure used
- Processing time, protocol
- Separation of blood from cells
- Centrifugation, speed and duration
- Aliquotting before analysis, handing and storage of those aliquots
- Time to analysis

Storage

- Snap frozen versus −20°C versus −80°C
- Time and temperature, before freezing
- Short- or long-term storage
- Storage temperature
- Storage materials
- Polystyrene versus polypropylene
- Number of freeze-thaw cycles

Data from Rai AJ, Gelfand CA, Haywood BC, et al. HUPO Plasma Proteome Project specimen collection and handling: towards the standardization of parameters for plasma proteome samples. Proteomics 2005;5:3262–77.

Box 2
Sample protocol successfully implemented in a clinical environment

I. Procedure: Serum

1. Fill 10 mL polypropylene (tube #1) right before skin incision

2. Invert tube several times, then leave upright at room temperature to clot for 1 hour

3. Centrifuge for 8 minutes at 3000 rpm

4. Transfer serum, the clear layer above the clot, in tube #2

5. Centrifuge for 8 minutes at 3000 rpm

6. Transfer serum in tube #3

7. Store immediately in −80°C freezer

II. Procedure: Plasma

1. Fill 5 mL polypropylene EDTA tube (tube #4) right before skin incision from central venous line

2. Invert tube several times, then process immediately

3. Centrifuge for 8 minutes at 3000 rpm

4. Transfer plasma into tube #5

5. Centrifuge for 8 minutes at 3000 rpm

6. Transfer supernatant (now platelet poor) into tube #5

7. Store immediately in −80°C freezer

   ↑ In the operating room

   ↓ In the laboratory

III. Serum: Aliquoting

1. Five tubes with 150 μL each

2. Remainder of serum should be distributed in 500-μL aliquotes

3. Cryovials tubes should be transferred to liquid nitrogen to snap freeze the serum and then transfer tubes to −80°C for storage

IV. Plasma: Aliquoting

1. Five tubes with 150 μL each

2. Remainder of plasma should be distributed in 500-μL aliquotes

3. Cryovials tubes should be transferred to liquid nitrogen to snap freeze the serum and then transfer tubes to −80°C for storage

V. Notes

1. It is extremely important to keep 1 hour clotting time consistent for serum samples

2. Always use the same brand of tubes

3. Avoid repeated freeze-thaw cycles

---

antibody-based validation techniques sometimes exhibit difficulty in correctly recognizing isoforms of posttranslational modifications. When there are no antibodies or recombinant proteins available, the researcher has to judge if the candidate marker justifies the cost and labor required to develop new and specific high-affinity antibodies. For this reason, the future of candidate marker validation might be in techniques that allow for antibody-independent quantitation.

Once a marker has been validated in the animal model or in pooled samples of the initial patient population, the marker has to be evaluated in a larger population with known and well-characterized phenotypes. This evaluation stage also collects information regarding the potential marker's stability, detectability, and release-clearance kinetics. Although many people are on the hunt for the "one and only" biomarker, and proteomics certainly has the potential to discover this marker, there are few examples of important, widely applied biomarkers that are the result of proteomic discovery. Most biomarkers that are broadly applied in clinical routines, such as cardiac troponin I or T (demonstrating diagnostic, therapeutic, and prognostic implications in cardiovascular disease), have matured over years and are the product of a specific biologic hypothesis.

The classic literature differentiates among three standard types of biomarker: type 0 (natural history marker); type 1 (drug activity); and type 2 (surrogate marker). Recent authors tend to use more functional designations: biomarkers that describe the risk of getting the disease (antecedent markers); screening biomarkers; biomarkers used to diagnose the disease; biomarkers that describe the levels of disease (staging); and prognostic markers. Prognostic markers include those that make a prediction regarding the natural course of the disease, but they may also predict response to therapy, recurrence rate, and efficacy of a therapy.[4,15,16]

Once a candidate marker has undergone validation within the initial patient population from which it was generated (ideally including the same samples), it must then be evaluated across a broader patient population. A common error is to move instead to an immediate comparison with a group of healthy controls. This is likely to yield highly significant results, but there is a substantial risk that identifications will be for very general markers of disease, such as an inflammatory process. The next step is to define normal and abnormal values; the most common method is to measure average values in the population, and then use the 95th, 97.5th or 99th percentile as a cutoff. Care has to be taken, however, because these discrimination limits in many cases define decision thresholds. Because many cases demonstrate a significant overlap between the general population and the patient population, it may be useful to establish longitudinal control values, meaning that each patient serves as his or her own control.

An important factor when judging biomarkers is considering, beyond sensitivity and specificity, the positive (or negative) predictive value of a marker. For example, although C-reactive protein might not be a very specific marker, unable to differentiate between pneumonia and rheumatoid arthritis, it does, if the patient is already diagnosed with pneumonia, provide valuable information about the progress of the disease and the response to therapy.

Whereas most clinicians tend to favor single biomarkers, and design their trials accordingly, researchers in the proteomics field largely believe that the future of biomarkers is in biomarker panels. Strictly speaking, the panel philosophy is not new. Every clinician would accept the fact that measuring creatinine in an oliguric patient does not yield sufficient information for an accurate diagnosis. Nevertheless, no clinician would exchange this marker for another one; they would rather order additional tests (and in so doing, effectively create their own biomarker panel). Predefined multimarker panels can enhance sensitivity and specificity compared with each marker alone. As an example, C-reactive protein and low-density lipoprotein are both markers for cardiovascular risk; but when combined, they consistently demonstrate higher predictive power than either by itself.

Multiplex assays represent a promising new strategy in cardiovascular diagnostics. As de novo proteomics analysis gets more and more streamlined, and robust high-throughput methods are developed, validation becomes the bottleneck for biomarker development. Multiplex assays allow the simultaneous assessment of several biomarkers within the same sample, greatly enhancing both the standardization and the accuracy of the validation. A successful multiplex assay requires less sample quantity, and is far more cost-effective, than a monoplex assay. But this approach only gains ground slowly in the clinical laboratory setting, because there are still obstacles to putting a set of clinically important biomarkers in a single multiplex assay. Recently, however, an alternative way of performing multiplex assays has arisen. Multiple reactions monitoring is a long-standing MS-based technique that has been used in the pharmaceutical industry for drug development and other small-molecule applications. Multiple reactions monitoring was recently introduced for peptides in complex mixtures (eg, plasma), with the possibility to perform quantitative, antibody-independent multiplexing where the abundance of peptides derived from a parent peptide is compared with a known amount of spiked-in peptide.[17] Although this is a very promising technique, antibody-based methods, such as sandwich assays, are currently the most common.

Creation of a meaningful assay requires a common theme, whether it is related to a certain pathologic condition (eg, heart failure) or a particular class of proteins (eg, cytokines). Because the plasma levels of secreted proteins span up to nine magnitudes, analytes must be selected based on their concentration. Most multiplex assays, for instance, cannot deal with the greater than 100-fold average difference expected between the analytes of healthy individuals and patients. After a set of potential analytes for multiplexing has been identified, each analyte must be optimized within a monoplex to establish a baseline. A crucial role is played by the diluent used to dilute the samples and antibodies. Although assays might perform very well with bovine serum albumin as a standard diluent, they might produce completely different results when a diluent resembling the more complex nature of the human serum is used. Contemporary multiplexes generally use one of two different strategies: a sandwich immunoassay, where the analyte is bound to a capture antibody printed onto a surface; or a single-antibody, direct-labeling assay. Multiplex platforms, such as Bio-Plex (Bio-Rad Laboratories, Hercules, California), use a detection antibody-labeled bead population, analyzed with a modified flow cytometer. Although this is an established platform, bead-based assays seem to require more hardware maintenance compared with other systems, and may be somewhat less ideal in a nonclinical setting, where the hardware is not used on a daily basis and quality checks are not rigorously performed. The authors prefer a platform with robust hardware that requires minimal maintenance, such as the Ruthenium-based multiplex platform Sector Imager (Mesoscale Discovery, Gaithersburg, Maryland). It is important to note that research and clinical applications may place different demands on assay platforms.

Reproducibility is critically important when deploying multiplex platforms in a clinical setting, even if they are not for direct diagnostic use. The authors consider results valid when (1) the recovery of the standards/calibrators is $100 \pm 20\%$ (recovery = expected concentration divided by calculated concentration multiplied by 100); (2) the coefficient of variation is less than 20% (CV% = standard deviation divided by the average of replicates multiplied by 100); (3) intra-assay CV is less than 10%; and (4) interassay CV is less than 20%. A full run is considered valid when greater than 85% of samples lie within these result specifications. At least for research use, transparency in any data analysis performed according to manufacturer's algorithms (eg, as a part of instrument operation) is imperative (**Fig. 3**). Otherwise, parameters like lowest level of detection and lowest level of quantification cannot be judged objectively. When results from different multiplex platforms have to be compared, the authors recommend exporting the raw data and analyzing it using commercially available software; this removes any

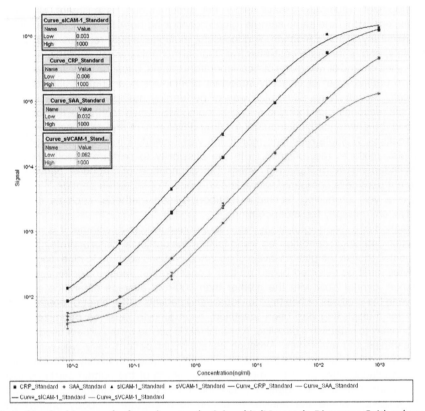

Fig. 3. Standard curves of a four-plex vascular injury kit (Mesoscale Discovery, Gaithersburg, Maryland), showing the sigmoidal dose-response curve typical of immunoassays.

differential between manufacturer's calculation parameters and ensures comparable results across the board.

The selection criteria used for candidate biomarkers can include such factors as the diagnostic window requirements, the extent of maximum change between control and disease population, overlap with other diseases, or lack of change caused by age or drugs. Some of the most promising biomarkers are present exclusively or extensively in diseased patients: cardiac troponin I and T, used for diagnosis of myocardial infarction, are great examples of such markers. These isoforms are highly abundant proteins in cardiac muscle, but are only present in minuscule quantities in the blood of patients without myocardial necrosis.[18–20] This situation led researchers to screen whole tissue samples (eg, heart) for candidate marker identification, and then move to easily accessible sample types (eg, serum-plasma or urine) for detection. This approach is appropriate for diseases where necrosis or cell leakage is a major factor. In other cases, however, protein biomarkers must arise from cellular secreted proteins or from proteins present on the cell membrane. B-natriuretic peptide (as a biomarker for heart failure) is an example of a secreted protein: it is present in healthy individuals, but the change in biomarker plasma levels over time, within the individual patient, is more important than the absolute value at any given time.

Cardiovascular disease is a systemic condition, and most patients do have other associated diseases, such as diabetes. Multiple disease markers, which are specific to different diseases, may be present in blood, confounding de novo discovery. If in the search for biomarkers researchers simply compare samples (eg, between patients with cardiovascular disease and healthy controls), any discovered marker could easily be for diabetes and not for cardiovascular disease. This is further complicated by the large numbers of initially promising biomarkers that turn out to be very general markers of disease, demonstrating only systemic, instead of disease-specific, involvement. Recent research estimates that only a small percentage of all proteins (about 4%) are truly cell-type specific.[21] It might not be the mere presence of a protein that makes the cell unique, but rather the amount of the protein in question. There is, at the same time, a strong case to be made that isoforms from the same protein can be products either of different genes (eg, fast skeletal troponin I versus cardiac troponin I) or of splice variants of the same gene. Disease-induced modifications of a protein, such as degradation products of cardiac troponin I, may have the ability to increase tissue specificity.[22–24]

PROTEOMICS AND CLINICAL PHYSICIAN PARTNERSHIPS

Successful proteomics studies require a team effort, a partnership. It is only after careful, joint review of the study protocol, with both a clinician and the proteomics scientist, that a proteomics study can be successfully launched. The clinician has to understand the demands and limits of the proteomics approach, not only in terms of sample

---

Box 3
Nongaseous emboli present in cardiopulmonary bypass circuit, potentially interfering with analysis using proteomics techniques

- Microthrombi (eg, fibrin)
- Platelet aggregates
- Red cell aggregates
- Denatured proteins
- Fat or lipids
- Cold-reacting antibodies
- Bone fragments
- Muscle fragments
- Calcium particles
- Cotton fibers
- Plastic particles
- Filter material
- Tubing fragments
- Metal
- Talc
- Thread
- Bone wax
- Microfibrillar collagen
- Silicone antifoam

quality but also regarding resource requirements (ie, time and money). The proteomics scientist must learn what is feasible within the clinical setting, and what disease-specific circumstances influence the analysis. For example, a proteomics scientist engaged in a promising study in renal failure should be eager to learn that the definition of the nephrotic syndrome is a protein loss through the kidneys of greater than 3 g/day: accurate representation requires that they normalize their results to total protein content, and this greatly influences the analysis compared with a control population. The same holds true with the analysis of blood from patients undergoing open heart surgery using cardiopulmonary bypass: the surgeon has to tell the scientist that they stopped the heart using high molar potassium solutions; that they primed the heart lung machine with exogenously supplied albumin; that they circulated the blood for 2 hours through plastic tubing; and that they counteracted the activation of the coagulation cascade with the use of aprotinin or tranexamic acid (**Box 3**).

The authors encourage the basic scientist, when working in the cardiovascular field, to spend a day with a cardiologist in the chest-pain unit or with a cardiac surgeon in the operating room, to get a feeling for how samples are won and what is really being done physically and functionally in the particular study. On the other side, clinicians are encouraged to listen carefully to the scientist when they describe the variety of factors influencing subsequent sample analysis. All of this collaborative preparation should happen before the first sample is taken. Additionally, most researchers seek statistical advice when planning a new study. Newcomers to the complex field of biomarker discovery should similarly consult with an established scientist to plan and carry out research that achieves meaningful results.

SUMMARY

Proteomics holds tremendous promise for the diagnosis, prognosis, and treatment of cardiovascular disease, and is already changing the way clinicians look at biomarkers of all kinds. But the field and techniques are complex and rigorous, and even in the most capable proteomics facilities, more significant biomarkers are passed over than discovered every day.

ACKNOWLEDGMENTS

We thank Shandev Rai for improving the manuscript with editorial comments and suggestions.

REFERENCES

1. Gerszten RE, Accurso F, Bernard GR, et al. Challenges in translating plasma proteomics from bench to bedside: update from the NHLBI Clinical Proteomics Programs. Am J Physiol Lung Cell Mol Physiol 2008;295:16–22.
2. Malmström J, Lee H, Aebersold R. Advances in proteomic workflows for systems biology. Curr Opin Biotechnol 2007;18:378–84.
3. Arrell DK, Neverova I, Van Eyk JE. Cardiovascular proteomics: evolution and potential. Circ Res 2001;88:763–73.
4. Jaffe AS, Babuin L, Apple FS. Biomarkers in acute cardiac disease: the present and the future. J Am Coll Cardiol 2006;48:1–11.
5. Vivanco F, Martín-Ventura JL, Duran MC, et al. Quest for novel cardiovascular biomarkers by proteomic analysis. J Proteome Res 2005;4:1181–91.
6. Stanley BA, Gundry RL, Cotter RJ, et al. Heart disease, clinical proteomics and mass spectrometry. Dis Markers 2004;20:167–78.

7. Arab S, Gramolini AO, Ping P, et al. Cardiovascular proteomics: tools to develop novel biomarkers and potential applications. J Am Coll Cardiol 2006;48:1733–41.
8. Parikh SV, de Lemos JA. Biomarkers in cardiovascular disease: integrating pathophysiology into clinical practice. Am J Med Sci 2006;332:186–97.
9. Matt P, Fu Z, Fu Q, et al. Biomarker discovery: proteome fractionation and separation in biological samples. Physiol Genomics 2008;33:12–7.
10. McDonald T, Sheng S, Stanley B, et al. Expanding the subproteome of the inner mitochondria using protein separation technologies: one- and two-dimensional liquid chromatography and two-dimensional gel electrophoresis. Mol Cell Proteomics 2006;5:2392–411.
11. Tammen H, Schulte I, Hess R, et al. Peptidomic analysis of human blood specimens: comparison between plasma specimens and serum by differential peptide display. Proteomics 2005;5:3414–22.
12. Arkin CF, Ernst DJ, Marler A, et al. Tubes and additives for venous blood specimen collection; approved standard. Fifth Edition. Wayne (PA): NCCLS; 2003.
13. Rai AJ, Gelfand CA, Haywood BC, et al. HUPO Plasma proteome project specimen collection and handling: towards the standardization of parameters for plasma proteome samples. Proteomics 2005;5:3262–77.
14. Matt P, Habashi J, Carrel T, et al. Recent advances in understanding Marfan syndrome: should we now treat surgical patients with losartan? J Thorac Cardiovasc Surg 2007;135:389–94.
15. Vasan RS. Biomarkers of cardiovascular disease: molecular basis and practical considerations. Circulation 2006;113:2335–62.
16. Anderson L. Candidate-based proteomics in the search for biomarkers of cardiovascular disease. J Physiol 2005;563:23–60.
17. Anderson L, Hunter CL. Quantitative mass spectrometric multiple reaction monitoring assays for major plasma proteins. Mol Cell Proteomics 2006;5:573–88.
18. Apple FS, Murakami MM. Serum and plasma cardiac troponin I 99th percentile reference values for 3 2nd-generation assays. Clin Chem 2007;53:1558–60.
19. Apple FS, Pearce LA, Doyle PJ, et al. Cardiac troponin risk stratification based on 99th percentile reference cutoffs in patients with ischemic symptoms suggestive of acute coronary syndrome: influence of estimated glomerular filtration rates. Am J Clin Pathol 2007;127:598–603.
20. Apple FS. Cardiac troponin monitoring for detection of myocardial infarction: newer generation assays are here to stay. Clin Chim Acta 2007;380:1–3.
21. Berglund L, Björling E, Oksvold P, et al. A genecentric human protein atlas for expression profiles based on antibodies. Mol Cell Proteomics 2008;10:2019–27.
22. Bovenkamp DE, Stanley BA, Van Eyk JE. Optimization of cardiac troponin I pulldown by IDM affinity beads and SELDI. Methods Mol Biol 2007;357:91–102.
23. Madsen LH, Christensen G, Lund T, et al. Time course of degradation of cardiac troponin I in patients with acute ST-elevation myocardial infarction: the ASSENT-2 troponin substudy. Circ Res 2006;99:1141–7.
24. McDonough JL, Van Eyk JE. Developing the next generation of cardiac markers: disease-induced modifications of troponin I. Prog Cardiovasc Dis 2004;47:207–16.

Clinical Proteomic Applications of Formalin-Fixed Paraffin-Embedded Tissues

Josip Blonder, MD, Timothy D. Veenstra, PhD*

KEYWORDS

- Clinical specimens • Mass spectrometry • Proteomics
- Formalin-fixed tissues • Biomarker discovery

There have been a number of exciting new events in the context of basic research over the past 10 to 15 years. One of the most recognizable developments is the conception and completion of the Human Genome Project, which enabled scientists to begin routinely studying thousands of genes and transcripts in single experiments.[1] Following suit, scientists began developing methods capable of characterizing thousands of proteins in a single experiment.[2] These burgeoning fields of genomics and proteomics do not represent the pinnacle because scientists are quickly developing metabolomics, a field in which comprehensive analysis of as many metabolites as possible in a single sample is the goal. There are at least two common threads that link these discovery-driven fields together: a group of visionary scientists with novel ideas, and developments in technology enabling these ideas to be tested.

For proteomics, the major technology development was coupling separation science with mass spectrometry (MS). Although both technologies have been around for several decades, it was not until the 1990s that investigators combined the separation capabilities of two-dimensional polyacrylamide gel electrophoresis with the ability to identify the resolved proteins using MS.[2,3] Since this time, different chromatographic and electrophoretic methods have been customized and even combined to optimize the fractionation of complex proteomic mixtures before their analysis by MS.[4] MS

This project has been funded in whole or in part with federal funds from the National Cancer Institute, National Institutes of Health, under Contract N01-CO-12400. The content of this publication does not necessarily reflect the views or policies of the Department of Health and Human Services, nor does mention of trade names, commercial products, or organization imply endorsement by the United States Government.

Laboratory of Proteomics and Analytical Technologies, SAIC-Frederick, National Cancer Institute at Frederick, 1050 Boyles Street, Frederick, MD 21702, USA

* Corresponding author.

E-mail address: veenstra@ncifcrf.gov (T.D. Veenstra).

Clin Lab Med 29 (2009) 101–113
doi:10.1016/j.cll.2009.01.006
0272-2712/09/$ – see front matter © 2009 Elsevier Inc. All rights reserved.

technology has seen exponential leaps in instrumental capability in almost every analytical parameter.[5] Modern spectrometers provide routine sensitivity into the high attomolar range; extremely high mass accuracy (eg, sub parts per million in specialized applications); and a rapid duty cycle of data-dependent acquisition mode enabling large numbers of peptides to be sequenced quickly. The combination of high-resolution liquid chromatography (LC) separations and high-performance MS has enabled thousands of proteins to be identified in biofluids, such as serum and plasma.[6]

THE MOVE TO CLINICAL SAMPLES

Many of the early technical developments, related to the ability to identify thousands of proteins in complex samples, were accomplished using proteomes extracted from simple organisms, such as *Escherichia coli* and yeast.[7,8] These initial studies demonstrated the necessity of state-of-the art sample preparation, chromatography, MS instrumentation, and bioinformatics to achieve comprehensive proteome coverage. Over the next couple of years much of the focus of these types of proteomic studies was on simple organisms or cells in culture to identify differentially expressed proteins when the systems were treated with some external perturbation.[9] The proteome-wide coverage attainable using LC-MS, however, brought a new potential use to this technology: the discovery of disease-specific biomarkers.

Experimental studies to discover biomarkers using high-throughput LC-MS methods used easily accessible patient samples, such as urine, serum, and plasma. There are many good reasons for choosing these samples, including the fact that they are acquired at most routine physicals and their molecular content can be reflective and indicative of the general health of the patient (eg, high cholesterol, excess protein in urine). The transition to biofluid analysis, however, was not as straightforward as anticipated, especially for the cases of serum and plasma. Both of these biofluids seem ideal for proteomic analysis because they have a very high protein concentration (in excess of 50 mg/mL). The problem, however, is that most of protein concentration in serum/ plasma is contributed by a single protein, albumin. This fact makes it necessary to remove this protein, along with other high abundant proteins, from serum/plasma before LC-MS analysis. Fortunately, depletion strategies have enabled this obstacle to be overcome and the number of proteins identifiable in serum-plasma has increased from a few hundred to a few thousand over the past 5 years.[6]

Even with this exponential analytical leap, the discovery of biomarkers in biofluids has remained elusive. Ask investigators to name a protein biomarker that has been discovered using proteomic technology in the recent past and most would struggle. Even the success in the discovery of the antiproliferative factor, a biomarker for interstitial cystitis, was more dependent on the availability of a cell-based activity-assay to monitor for the presence of this protein than the actual final MS identification.[10] This lack of real success has made the entire field re-evaluate the strategy of using biofluids as the matrix from which to find disease-specific protein biomarkers. However, the discovery of a biomarker in a biofluid, such as urine, serum, or plasma, would be ideal because these samples are easily acquired without causing any discomfort to the patient. Detecting novel biomarkers in these matrices, however, presents an intricate task.[11] First, a biomarker is expected to have its peak concentration directly at the site of the tumor. Its concentration would likely decrease by several orders of magnitude by dilution effect as it moves through the circulatory system and is either naturally expelled from the body or is acquired through a blood draw. Second, the circulatory system is rich in proteases that could dramatically change the character of any potential biomarker before its acquisition for analysis. Third, even if a potentially useful biomarker is found during the analysis of a series of comparative biofluid samples, it can be extremely difficult to show conclusively that its differential abundance was caused by solely, or even primarily, the presence of the tumor.

These challenges have made a number of investigators turn toward tissues. There are a number of advantages in analyzing tissues. First, the concentration of any potential tissue-derived biomarker is expected to be at its peak at the site of the pathologic process. Second, the concentration of that biomarker can be compared with that within the surrounding cells and tissue. Third, mechanistic studies can be done to determine if the biomarker plays any functional role in the progression of the tumor. Analyzing tissues, however, has one fundamental disadvantage: sample acquisition. Acquiring tumor and tissue samples is highly invasive and it is simply difficult to obtain large numbers of specimen from either disease-affected patients or healthy tissue from matched controls.

THE MOVEMENT TO FORMALIN-FIXED PARAFFIN-EMBEDDED TISSUES

Although it would be a great opportunity to obtain samples prospectively from patients, this difficulty has not prevented investigators from exploring novel sources of tissues. There already exists an enormous cohort of almost every conceivable tumor in the form of formalin-fixed paraffin-embedded (FFPE) tissue. This method of storing tissue has existed for decades and large repositories containing libraries of FFPE tissue blocks exist in essentially every major medical center worldwide.[12] Immunohistochemistry (IHC) has been applied to FFPE tissues for a number of years and has been invaluable to pathologists, increasing their ability to accurately stratify tumors. The application of IHC to FFPE tissues has required a number of important technology developments over the past 30 years to make it an invaluable diagnostic tool.[13,14] These developments include increasingly sensitive detection systems and several pretreatments before antibody immunostaining so that the antigens that are modified by formalin fixation can be recovered. Many of the early antigen retrieval methods, such as enzymatic digestion, did not provide satisfactory results for many antigens. The search for a simple and effective retrieval method has become a hot topic in IHC since the early 1970s.[15] The method of boiling paraffin tissue sections in water, known as "high temperature–heating antigen retrieval," was shown almost two decades ago to improve IHC staining possible on FFPE tissues.[14] This technique has become accepted and used by pathologists in clinical laboratories worldwide and functions as a simple and effective method to achieve satisfactory immunostaining on archival tissue sections.[16] Although IHC is extremely valuable, it requires foreknowledge of the protein of interest and does not permit the finding of novel protein markers of disease without an risky/tedious trial and error approach. It would be invaluable to analyze FFPE tissues using modern technology and discovery-based proteomic approaches where the aim is to identify novel proteins that can be used to characterize diseases better, such as cancer at the site of pathological process.

Considering their common availability, why have FFPE tissues not been used in these types of proteomic studies until very recently? There are two main reasons. One is simply related to the limited amount of protein that can be extracted from FFPE tissue sections and the other is related to their formalin-caused cross-linking. MS is the analytical method of choice for discovery-based proteomic studies, and there is a direct correlation between the number of proteins that can be identified in a complex mixture (eg, a tissue section) and the amount of material available. When using tissue sections, the amount of protein available is on the order of 5 to 25 μg depending on the size of the section and whether laser capture microdissection is used to harvest specific cells. Fortunately, recent developments in MS technology[17] have enabled hundreds of proteins to be identified confidently using this small amount of material. Although this number is far from what is anticipated to be within any complex proteome, it still provides sufficient coverage to find potential differences between tumorous and healthy cells. The second reason is related to the effects of the formalin-related chemical cross-links that bind and fix biomolecules within the cell. Several years ago, a group evaluated the ability to extract intact proteins from FFPE tissue for proteomic analysis.[18] In this study, they attempted to separate the intact proteins using two-dimensional polyacrylamide gel electrophoresis before MS analysis. After staining, the resultant gel showed essentially no resolved protein spots. They correctly concluded that FFPE tissue was intractable to proteomic analysis using this method scheme because of the inherent intracovalent and intercovalent cross-links between proteins and other biomolecules. Although this study did not find FFPE tissues useful, this group should be credited for the recognition of the potential value of this material for discovery-based proteomic studies. Fortunately, investigators have found a method that does not require reversal of the formalin cross-links to characterize proteomes extracted from FFPE tissues. This method takes advantage of the fact that MS actually analyzes peptides generated by tryptic digestion of proteins, rather than analyzing the intact proteins. Using this subtle fact enables MS identification of non–cross-linked tryptic peptides, whereas peptides modified by the fixation process are ignored in the proteomic comparisons.

APPLICATION OF FORMALIN-FIXED PARAFFIN-EMBEDDED TISSUES FOR PROTEOMIC DISCOVERY

One of the earliest applications showing the use of conducting global characterization of proteomes extracted from FFPE tissue using MS was published in 2005.[19] In this study, a single whole-mount tissue section was cut from a FFPE prostate tissue obtained from a radical prostatectomy. Pathohistologic analysis of this section displayed regions of prostatic carcinoma, well (WD), moderately (MD), and poorly (PD) (5%) differentiated. Immunohistochemistry was initially used to identify tissue regions that expressed prostate-specific antigen (PSA), a known marker for prostate cancer. Standard hematoxylin and eosin staining of the whole-mount tissue section revealed tumor regions (PCa), a region of benign prostatic hyperplasia (BPH), and a stromal region. The IHC analysis revealed that the tumor and BPH regions stained positive for PSA, whereas the stromal region was negative. Once the regions of PCa, BPH, and stroma were defined, laser capture microdissection was used to acquire approximately 200,000 cells from the PCA and BPH regions of the tissue section (**Fig. 1**). These cells were then separately lysed in the presence of trypsin to reduce the intact proteins into tryptic peptides. The resultant peptides were analyzed directly using reversed-phase liquid chromatography coupled directly on-line with MS. Because the proteins are digested into peptides, two-dimensional polyacrylamide gel electrophoresis cannot be used effectively to fractionate the proteome. Over 1300 and 2200 unique, fully tryptic (unmodified) peptides representing 702 and 1156 unique proteins were identified in the BPH and PCa FFPE tissue extracts, respectively. The number of peptides identified for each protein was used as a rough indicator of a protein's relative abundance in PCa and BPH cells. Because of the limited amount of starting material, the proteins that were identified by the greatest number of peptides were members of the highly abundant cytoskeletal protein family (ie, actin, collagen, myosin, and so forth). Several known prostate cancer markers, such as PSA and prostatic acid phosphatase, however, were identified by multiple unique peptides. Unfortunately, each of these proteins was identified at roughly equal levels in both PCa and BPH cells. An

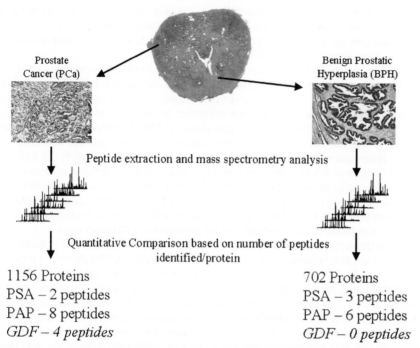

Peptide extraction and mass spectrometry analysis

Quantitative Comparison based on number of peptides
identified/protein

1156 Proteins

PSA – 2 peptides

PAP – 8 peptides

GDF – 4 peptides

702 Proteins

PSA – 3 peptides

PAP – 6 peptides

GDF – 0 peptides

Fig.1. Global proteomic analysis of prostate cancer and benign prostatic hyperplasia cells obtained from a FFPE prostate tissue using laser capture microdissection. In this analysis, over 1100 and 700 proteins were identified from the PCa and BPH cells, respectively. Although a number of PCa-related proteins, such as prostate specific antigen (PSA) and prostatic acid phosphatase (PAP), were identified, their levels in the two cell types were not appreciatively different. Growth differentiation factor 15 (GDF-15), however, was identified only in the PCa cells.

interesting finding was that growth differentiation factor 15 was identified by four unique peptides in the PCa cell proteome, whereas no peptides originating from this protein were identified in the proteome extracted from BPH cells. A recent study has shown that serum growth differentiation factor 15 can function as an independent marker of the presence of PCa[20] confirming the potential application of this protein as a biomarker.

VALIDATION OF GLOBAL COMPARATIVE STUDIES IS CRITICAL

Once it became clear that meaningful proteomic results could be obtained from FFPE tissues, a number of different studies examining these clinical samples were completed. Although all of these studies showed the ability to find differences between comparative tissues or cell types, the accuracy and precision of the quantitative measurements provided were insufficient to have absolute confidence in the differences observed solely by using the number of peptides identified for each protein using MS. Quantitative analysis of FFPE tissue sections using this LC-MS method is not suitable for clinical analysis because of a number of factors including throughput, accuracy, and precision. These global comparative studies essentially provide possibilities of actual protein abundance differences and any potential difference requires orthogonal validation. The true value in global discovery studies, however, is that they are able to provide useful information that has a significant probability of being confirmed in subsequent validation studies. Once potentially valuable protein markers can be discovered, a number of proteins can be validated across a large number of tissue sections using much higher-throughput methods.

This phenomenon is illustrated in a study that uses FFPE tissue sections obtained from PD, MD, and WD head and neck squamous cell carcinoma tumors.[21] In this study, laser capture microdissection was used to extract cells from normal squamous epithelial tissue and tumors that were classified as PD, MD, or WD. In each case approximately 20,000 cells were analyzed using LC-MS. As with the example shown previously, the number of peptides identified per individual protein was used as a crude quantitative measurement of a protein's relative abundance in the four cell types. A number of differences were seen between the cells, and in particular cytokeratin 4 was found to be more abundant in normal epithelial tissue compared with tumor cells, whereas three proteins (cytokeratin 16, vimentin, and desmoplakin) were found to be more abundant in the tumor cells compared with normal epithelial tissue. Desmoplakin was found to be particularly more abundant in WD tumor cells.

With the discovery of potential markers of head and neck squamous cell carcinoma, the next (absolutely necessary) step was orthogonal validation. The discovery process using MS is slow and can require almost 1 week per sample; fortunately, once the potential markers are identified, the validation methods (eg, immunoassays) that are available allow a number of different tissue sections to be tested concurrently. In this study, archival tissues consisting of normal epithelial and tumor head and neck squamous cell carcinoma were processed and used for immunodetection of the indicated proteins with appropriate antibodies against cytokeratin 4, vimentin, and desmoplakin (**Fig. 2**). The IHC validation was performed using a tissue microarray (TMA), which permits multiple tissue slides to be processed concurrently. For each antibody tested, 10 normal tissue sections were used, whereas for the PD, MD, and WD tumors between 33 and 105 tissues were analyzed. In **Fig. 2** representative TMA results for the three proteins are shown at the top. Individually stained tissues were scored based on tissue differentiation and the intensity of staining by each individual antibody. For cytokeratin 4, light gray represents greater than 5% and less than 25% of cells within the section stained; mid gray, 26% to 50% of the cells stained; dark gray, 51% to 75% of the cells stained; and black, 76% to 100% of the cells stained. The results show that almost all of the cells in the normal tissues were immunopositive for vimentin, whereas very few of the tumor cells showed staining for this protein. For vimentin and desmoplakin, the percentage of positive tumors for each stage of differentiation (spotted box) compared with negative (white box) is depicted. None of the 10 normal tissues stained for vimentin showed positive immunoreactivity, whereas approximately 60% to 70% of the tumors showed positive staining for this protein. For desmoplakin, all of the tissues were immunoreactive for this protein, whereas approximately 5% to 15% of the tumors were negative. In each case, the number of normal (nonneoplastic) tissues analyzed was 10, and the number of head and neck squamous cell carcinoma cancer tissues is indicated at the top of each bar.

QUANTITATIVE ANALYSIS OF SPECIFIC PROTEINS IN FORMALIN-FIXED PARAFFIN-EMBEDDED TISSUES

At about the same time, a group led by Dr. David Han at the University of Connecticut independently developed a similar method to extract peptides from FFPE tissue sections for global characterization using MS.[22] This study, also using FFPE prostate cancer tissue samples, was able to identify 428 prostate-expressed proteins using

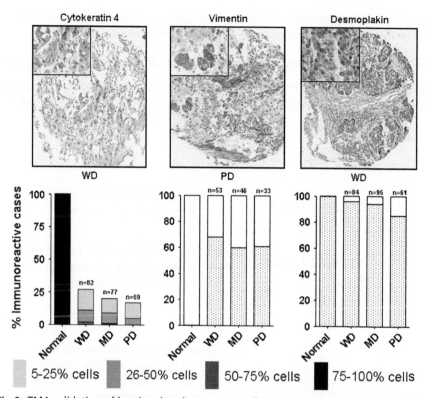

Fig. 2. TMA validation of head and neck squamous cell carcinoma biomarkers identified by global proteomic analysis of well- (WD), moderately (MD), and poorly differentiated (PD) head and neck squamous cell carcinoma tumor samples. The upper panel shows representative TMA cores stained for cytokeratin 16, vimentin, and desmoplakin using IHC. The stained TMAs were "scored" based on tissue differentiation and intensity of IHC staining. For cytokeratin 4, light gray represents >5% and <25%; mid gray, 26% to 50%; dark gray, 51% to 75%; and black, 76% to 100% of the cells stained positively for this protein. The scoring for vimentin and desmoplakin was based on the percentage of positive tumors for each stage of differentiation (*checkered box*) compared with negative (*white box*). In each case, the number of normal (ie, nonneoplastic) tissues analyzed was 10, and the number of head and neck squamous cell carcinoma cancer tissues is indicated above each column.

MS. Instead of conducting a global comparison between different cell types in the tissue, this group used a method that targets specific proteins for quantitation. This method (**Fig. 3**), termed AQUA (for absolute quantification), adds a known amount of a stable isotope-labeled peptide standard directed to a specific sequence in the protein of interest. An obvious candidate for this quantitation measurement was PSA. To quantify PSA in the prostate cancer tissue, a standard peptide (LSEPAELT-DAVK) was synthesized using heavy-isotope-containing amino acids. One hundred femtomole of this standard peptide was added to the tryptic digested FFPE tissue sections and the amount of PSA was quantified in five normal controls and in 15 cancerous prostate tissues (including low-, medium-, and high-grade cancers). The range of PSA quantified directly from various prostate and normal tissue sections was 0.5 to 140 pg. These results demonstrate the ability to target specific biomarkers, such as PSA, for the purpose of accurately quantitating their levels in FFPE tissues and potentially increasing the specificity and sensitivity in prostate cancer detection. The gain of this method compared with IHC is that it can provide an absolute concentration of PSA allowing accurate comparison across an infinite number of tumors.

APPLICATION OF TISSUE MICROARRAYS FOR FORMALIN-FIXED PARAFFIN-EMBEDDED TISSUES

One of the most exciting clinical proteomic applications of FFPE involves their use in TMA.[23–25] IHC is a fundamental diagnostic technique in modern clinical pathology and

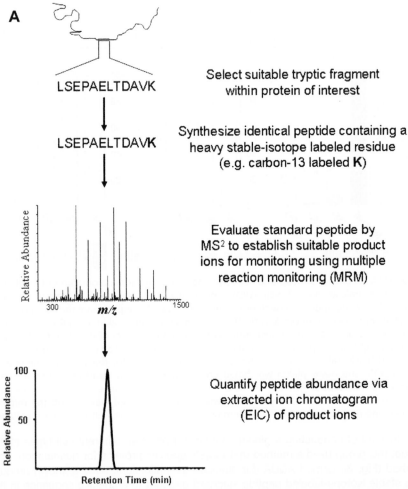

A

LSEPAELTDAVK

Select suitable tryptic fragment within protein of interest

LSEPAELTDAV**K**

Synthesize identical peptide containing a heavy stable-isotope labeled residue (e.g. carbon-13 labeled **K**)

Relative Abundance

300   *m/z*   1500

Evaluate standard peptide by MS^2 to establish suitable product ions for monitoring using multiple reaction monitoring (MRM)

Relative Abundance

100

50

Retention Time (min)

Quantify peptide abundance via extracted ion chromatogram (EIC) of product ions

Fig. 3. Absolute quantification of target protein within FFPE tissue section. (*A*) The first step in measuring the absolute quantity of a specific protein from a FFPE tissue is to select a tryptic peptide that acts as a surrogate for the whole protein. A synthesized version of this peptide containing a single heavy isotope-labeled amino acid is prepared and analyzed by MS^2 to find product ions of good intensity that allow unambiguous identification of the peptide. The concentration of the peptide is then correlated to the intensity of its peak obtained from an EIC. (*B*) To quantitate the protein in FFPE tissue samples, a known amount of the heavy isotope-labeled peptide is added to a solution containing the tissue sample, and the entire mixture is digested with trypsin. Analysis of the solution by MS^2 and comparison of the peak areas obtained from the EICs of the endogenous and internal standard peptide allows the absolute amount of target protein to be calculated.

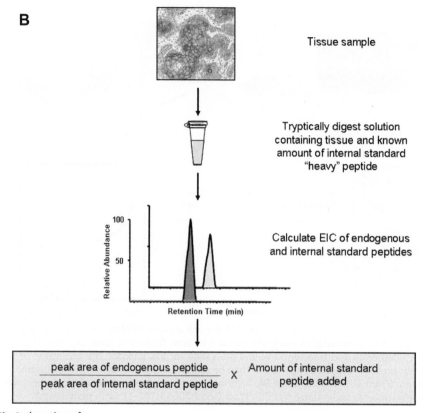

B

Tissue sample

Tryptically digest solution containing tissue and known amount of internal standard "heavy" peptide

Calculate EIC of endogenous and internal standard peptides

$$\frac{\text{peak area of endogenous peptide}}{\text{peak area of internal standard peptide}} \quad \text{X} \quad \begin{array}{c}\text{Amount of internal standard} \\ \text{peptide added}\end{array}$$

Fig. 3. (*continued*)

is a standard research tool in translational research laboratories. Instead of conducting IHCs on a single tissue at a time, TMAs allow for the concurrent analysis of tens to hundreds of specimens of tissue on a single slide. Other groups previously combined samples from different specimens on a single slide[26,27]; however, the TMA allows assessment in a more standardized way that minimizes the variability and definitely increases the throughput of IHC. In the construction of a TMA, archived FFPE tissues are used and specific regions of interest are cored from each tumor block (**Fig. 4**). These cores are typically 0.6 to 2 mm in diameter. The resultant core is then sectioned into thin slices, which are then transferred onto a glass slide for automated IHC analysis. The results of the IHC analysis can be assessed either manually or by automation and these data then linked to other available clinical data, - allowing better prediction of patient outcome. The advantage of TMAs is the high degree of precision and throughput that it provides for the analysis of these clinically important samples.

Although the effectiveness of IHC of FFPE tissues is becoming increasingly automated, it is still primarily used to measure a single protein at a time. The resolution of localizing the antigen is limited, because of the chromogenic substrate precipitate and thickness (3–4 μm) of the sections imaged in the light microscope. Chromogenic systems also saturate easily, rendering semiquantitative measurements less accurate.[28] Immunofluorescence, however, is capable of labeling multiple proteins through the use of different fluorophores and provides higher resolution because the fluorophores are directly conjugated to the antibody. Although immunofluorescence has

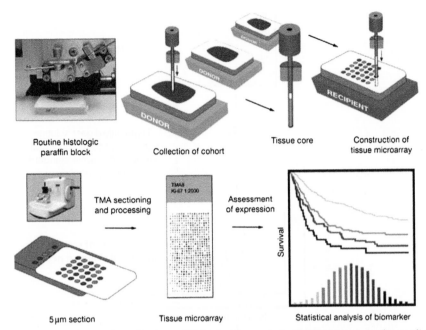

Fig. 4. Construction and application of TMA for the analysis of FFPE tissues. In the application of TMA, representative areas of interest are cored from FFPE tissue sections. The core is then sectioned and transferred onto a glass slide for IHC analysis. The expression of the specific proteins assayed using IHC can then be assessed either manually or in an automated fashion. (*From* Giltnane JM, Rimm DL. Technology insight: identification of biomarkers with tissue microarray technology. Nat Clin Pract Oncol 2004;1:104–11; with permission.)

been applied to cyrosections, it has not been often used for FFPE tissues. In recent years, there have been a number of reports describing the immunofluorescence labeling of FFPE;[30] however, they have not been widely used. Recently, Robertson and colleagues[28] developed and applied an immunofluorescence labeling approach to FFPE tissue that couples antigen retrieval, indirect immunofluorescence, and confocal laser scanning microscopy for imaging. An example provided in **Fig. 5** shows the labeling of cytokeratin 8/18, vimentin, and the estrogen receptor within single FFPE tissues. In addition, 4'-6-diamidino-2-phenylindole staining was also used for location of nicleai within the individual cells. In this example, normal breast tissue, breast tissue with columnar cell change, and both ductal carcinoma in situ and invasive components of an estrogen receptor positive breast cancer were analyzed. The advantage of multiple labeling is demonstrated in the observation that in normal breast tissue, estrogen receptor expression is limited to a subset of cytokeratin 8/18–positive luminal epithelial cells. In addition, multicolor visualization reveals that vimentin expression is restricted to the intralobular and interlobular stromal fibroblasts and vasculature. There is also low-level staining for vimentin in the myoepithelial cells; however, scattered vimentin-positive, cytokeratin 8/18–negative cells admixed with neoplastic cells can be found in high-grade ductal carcinoma in situ. The ability to semiquantitatively visualize multiple proteins within single tissue sections allows the pathologist rapidly to determine protein biomarker relationships within clinical tissue sections. This complex analysis also permits correlation between proteins involved in signaling pathways to be measured.

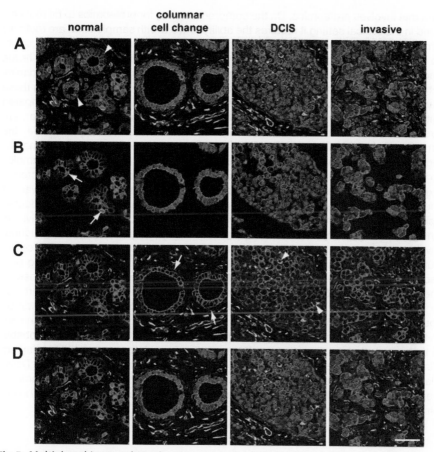

Fig. 5. Multiplexed immunohistochemistry analysis of FFPE tissue sections. Expression of cytokeratin (Ck) 8/18, estrogen receptor (ER), and vimentin in normal human breast and breast cancer. FFPE sections of human adult breast containing both normal tissue and columnar cell change, and an ER-positive breast cancer showing areas of ductal carcinoma in situ (DCIS) and invasive ductal carcinoma were stained using antibodies directed against Ck 8/18, vimentin, and ER. Nuclei are counterstained blue using DAPI. The colors in the figures represent the following: Ck 8/18 (*green*), ER (*red*), and vimentin (*yellow*). (*A*) Four-color images, arrowheads indicate Ck 8/18–negative myoepithelial cells. (*B*) Ck 8/18 and ER imaging with the arrows highlighting ER expression in luminal epithelial cells with concurrent high Ck 8/18 expression in normal breast cells. (*C*) Immunofluorescent imaging of Ck 8/18 and vimentin, with arrows highlighting vimentin expression in the myoepithelial cells of columnar cell change and arrowheads showing vimentin-positive, Ck 8/18–negative cells within the DCIS. (*D*) Ck 8/18, ER, and vimentin immunofluorescent staining in breast tissue. Scale bar, 50 μm. (*From* Robertson D, Savage K, Reis-Filho JS, et al. Multiple immunofluorescence labelling of formalin-fixed paraffin-embedded (FFPE) tissue. BMC Cell Biol 2008;9:13–22; with permission.)

SUMMARY AND FUTURE DIRECTIONS

One of the goals of proteomic researchers is to develop MS methods that can be used in clinical settings for the diagnosis or monitoring of disease progression.[6] To make this goal a reality significant compromise and strategic planning is required on the part that involves proteomics. On the compromise side, for proteomics to be routinely used in the clinical setting it requires the ability to work with samples that are routinely procured and analyzed within conventional clinical framework. This means the ability to routinely analyze clinical specimens including serum, plasma, urine, and tissue sections (both FFPE and frozen) customarily collected during outpatient or in-hospital interventions. Not only do methods need to continue developing for analyzing these samples, but they should also be optimized for limited amounts of sample compared with what is routinely used in a research setting. Tissue samples, in particular, are precious and difficult to obtain. Although FFPE tissues are widely available, the amount of material that can be routinely collected from them is limited. Fortunately, significant inroads have been made in the past few years in marrying clinical samples to MS[29] and other types of proteomic analysis methods[23] and this trend is expected to expand. On the strategic planning side, proteomic investigators need to be aware of the throughput required for clinical analysis. Almost all proteomic analyses conducted using MS are done on a one-sample per experiment basis. In addition, an individual analysis requires on the order of several minutes to hours to complete. This throughput level is not going to be sufficient for use in large clinical centers that may require hundreds of samples to be analyzed per day. Based on data obtained using proteomics as discovery tool, after validation, well-established affinity-based analysis methods, such as ELISA, can analyze and provide the results for hundreds of samples in a matter of hours. It is highly improbable that large-scale MS methods will be routinely used for global characterization of FFPE tissues in the clinical environment in the near future without a major leap in LC-MS technology. What is more probable is that assays that measure the absolute quantity of novel disease-related biomarkers discovered in global studies are applied in clinical laboratories. As shown by David Han's efforts,[22] such assays can be potentially developed to analyze tens of samples per day easily with a single MS instrument and eliminate much of the subjectivity in the stratification of tumors.

REFERENCES

1. Venter JC, Adams MD, Myers EW, et al. The sequence of the human genome. Science 2001;291:1304–51.
2. Wilkins MR, Sanchez JC, Gooley AA, et al. Progress with proteome projects: why all proteins expressed by a genome should be identified and how to do it. Biotechnol Genet Eng Rev 1996;13:19–50.
3. Muller EC, Thiede B, Zimny-Arndt U, et al. High-performance human myocardial two-dimensional electrophoresis database: edition 1996. Electrophoresis 1996; 17:1700–12.
4. Fournier ML, Gilmore JM, Martin-Brown SA, et al. Multidimensional separations-based shotgun proteomics. Chem Rev 2007;107:3654–86.
5. Zhou M, Veenstra TD. Mass spectrometry: m/z 1983-2008. Biotechniques 2008; 44:667–70.
6. Issaq HJ, Xiao Z, Veenstra TD. Serum and plasma proteomics. Chem Rev 2007; 107:3601–20.
7. Washburn MP, Wolters D, Yates III JR. Large-scale analysis of the yeast proteome by multidimensional protein identification technology. Nat Biotechnol 2001;19: 242–7.
8. Wu CC, MacCoss MJ. Shotgun proteomics: tools for the analysis of complex biological systems. Curr Opin Mol Ther 2002;4:242–50.

9. Lipton MS, Pasa-Tolic L, Anderson GA, et al. Global analysis of the *Deinococcus radiodurans* proteome by using accurate mass tags. Proc Natl Acad Sci U S A 2002;99:11049–54.

10. Keay SK, Szekely Z, Conrads TP, et al. An antiproliferative factor for interstitial cystitis patients is a frizzled 8 protein-related sialoglycopeptide. Proc Natl Acad Sci U S A 2004;101:11803–8.

11. Prieto DA, Ye X, Veenstra TD. Proteomic analysis of traumatic brain injury: the search for biomarkers. Expert Rev Proteomics 2008;5:283–91.

12. Wilkinson EJ, Hendricks JB. Role of the pathologist in biomarker studies. J Cell Biochem Suppl 1995;23:10–8.

13. Shi SR, Cote RJ, Taylor CR. Antigen retrieval techniques: current perspectives. J Histochem Cytochem 2001;49:931–8.

14. Shi SR, Key ME, Kalra KL. Antigen retrieval in formalin-fixed, paraffin-embedded tissues: an enhancement method for immunohistochemical staining based on microwave oven heating of tissue sections. J Histochem Cytochem 1991;39:741–8.

15. Taylor CR, Cote RJ. Immunomicroscopy: a diagnostic tool for the surgical pathologist. 2nd edition Philadelphia, WB Saunders; 1994.

16. Yamashita S. Heat-induced antigen retrieval: mechanisms and application to histochemistry. Prog Histochem Cytochem 2007;41:141–200.

17. Zhou M, Veenstra TD. Mass spectrometry: m/z 1983-2008. Biotechniques 2008; 71:61–70.

18. Ahram M, Flaig MJ, Gillespie JW, et al. Evaluation of ethanol-fixed, paraffin-embedded tissues for proteomic analysis. Proteomics 2003;3:413–21.

19. Hood BL, Darfler MM, Guiel TG, et al. Proteomic analysis of formalin-fixed prostate cancer tissue. Mol Cell Proteomics 2005;4:1741–53.

20. Nakamura T, Scorilas A, Stephan C, et al. Quantitative analysis of macrophage inhibitory cytokine-1 (MIC-1) gene expression in human prostatic tissues. Br J Cancer 2003;88:1101–4.

21. Patel V, Hood BL, Molinolo AA, et al. Proteomic analysis of laser-captured paraffin-embedded tissues: a molecular portrait of head and neck cancer progression. Clin Cancer Res 2008;14:1002–14.

22. Swang SI, Thumar J, Lundgren DH, et al. Direct cancer tissue proteomics: a method to identify candidate biomarkers from formalin-fixed paraffin-embedded archival tissues. Oncogene 2007;26:65–76.

23. Kononen J, Bubendorf L, Kallioniemi A, et al. Tissue microarrays for high-throughput molecular profiling of tumor specimens. Nat Med 1998;4:844–7.

24. Speer R, Wulfkuhle J, Espina V, et al. Development of reverse phase protein microarrays for clinical applications and patient-tailored therapy. Cancer Genomics Proteomics 2007;4:157–64.

25. Takikita M, Chung JY, Hewitt SM. Tissue microarrays enabling high-throughput molecular pathology. Curr Opin Biotechnol 2007;18:318–25.

26. Battifora H, Mehta P. The checkerboard tissue block: an improved multitissue control block. Lab Invest 1990;63:722–4.

27. Giltnane JM, Rimm DL. Technology insight: identification of biomarkers with tissue microarray technology. Nat Clin Pract Oncol 2004;1:104–11.

28. Robertson D, Savage K, Reis-Filho JS, et al. Multiple immunofluorescence labelling of formalin-fixed paraffin-embedded (FFPE) tissue. BMC Cell Biol 2008;9: 13–22.

29. Bataille F, Troppmann S, Klebl F, et al. Multiparameter immunofluorescence on paraffin-embedded tissue sections. Appl Immunohistochem Mol Morphol 2006; 14:225–8.

Development of High-Throughput Mass Spectrometry – Based Approaches for Cancer Biomarker Discovery and Implementation

Brian L. Hood, PhD[a,b], Nicolas A.S. Stewart, PhD[c],
Thomas P. Conrads, PhD[a,b,d],*

KEYWORDS

- Biomarker • Proteomics • Mass spectrometry
- Discovery • Validation

Armed with sequence information of the human and mouse genomes, a major aim of biological science is toward unraveling the underlying molecular events that lead to cellular function/dysfunction in disease, with the goal of discovering better diagnostic markers and therapeutic targets. Proteomics aims to facilitate this process by applying newly developed methods and advanced analytic tools, such as mass spectrometry (MS), for the investigation of the protein complement en masse. Proteomics is the comprehensive study of proteins, analyzing their structure, function, modifications, expression, interactions, and localization in complex biologic systems. The information obtained can help elucidate the function of individual proteins and establish the composition of functional units, protein–protein interactions, and dysregulated protein pathways and networks. Because proteins represent the preponderance of the

This work was supported by funds from the Department of Defense (PC074313), the Hillman Foundation, and the David Scaife Foundation.

[a] Clinical Proteomics Facility, University of Pittsburgh Cancer Institute, University of Pittsburgh School of Medicine, 204 Craft Avenue, Pittsburgh, PA 15213, USA
[b] Magee-Womens Research Institute, Suite B447, 204 Craft Avenue, Pittsburgh, PA 15213, USA
[c] Center for Clinical Pharmacology, Department of Medicine, University of Pittsburgh School of Medicine, 204 Craft Avenue, Pittsburgh, PA 15213, USA
[d] Department of Pharmacology & Chemical Biology, University of Pittsburgh Cancer Institute, University of Pittsburgh School of Medicine, 204 Craft Avenue, Pittsburgh, PA 15213, USA
* Corresponding author. Magee-Womens Research Institute, Suite B401, 204 Craft Avenue, Pittsburgh, PA, USA.
E-mail address: conradstp@upmc.edu (T.P. Conrads).

Clin Lab Med 29 (2009) 115–138
doi:10.1016/j.cll.2009.01.007
0272-2712/09/$ – see front matter © 2009 Elsevier Inc. All rights reserved.

biologically active molecules responsible for most cellular functions, it is critical to develop and apply technologies for conducting direct measurements of proteins that may be involved in cellular dysfunction underlying carcinogenesis. Proteomics is a leading-edge research technology that shows promise for revolutionizing the detection of cancer at an early stage, its molecular classification, and the assessment of patients' responses to treatments. In the clinical application of biomarkers, which has been referred to collectively as "theranostics," proteomic technologies offer considerable promise for providing prognostic information on individual patients, determining which patients will benefit most from a given therapy, providing improved and early assessment of individual patients' responses to therapy, identifying patients who can be treated effectively with minimally toxic therapies, identifying potential new drug targets, and enhancing the understanding of the therapeutic mode of action.

To be successful in discovery-driven applications of proteomics for cancer biomarker identification, advanced analytic and bioinformatic technologies are necessary. It is equally important that integrated strategies (**Fig. 1**) be devised that take advantage of the merits of model systems, such as cell lines or genetically engineered animal models, and clinically derived samples, such as tissues and biofluids, to maximize the wealth of information from these discovery efforts. Although the present article focuses on selected examples of the application of MS for proteomic biomarker discovery, it should be noted that MS-based proteomics is only one component of an ever-increasing suite of analytic tools and techniques that must be applied to gain a comprehensive, systems-level view of carcinogenesis. It is increasingly clear that the goal of personalized medicine will be realized only if investigators are successful in developing integrated approaches for interrogating carcinogenesis using genomics,

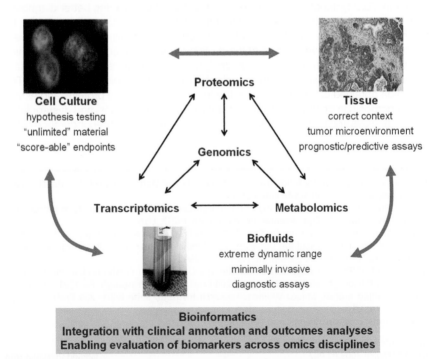

Fig. 1. Integrated sampling strategy for cancer biomarker discovery.

proteomics, and metabolomics and in deploying advanced bioinformatic strategies to explicate the molecular basis of cancer.

INTRODUCTION OF MASS SPECTROMETRY–BASED PROTEOMIC METHODOLOGIES

Two primary MS workflows are presently used to identify proteins on a proteome-wide scale (**Fig. 2**). The perhaps more classic method relies on the resolution of a complex mixture of proteins by two-dimensional polyacrylamide gel electrophoresis (2D-PAGE). In a 2D-PAGE experiment, complex protein mixtures are resolved in the first dimension by isoelectric focusing and in a second dimension by their molecular mass driven by electrophoresis through a polyacrylamide matrix. The resolved proteins can be visualized in the gel by a variety of stains including Coomassie blue, silver, or Sypro ruby. To detect differences among protein samples, each proteome sample is resolved in discrete gels and stained; the spot patterns and intensities are compared visually or computationally. Those protein "spots" of interest (eg, whose abundances differ) can be excised and enzymatically or chemically digested, and the resulting peptides can be analyzed by MS for identification. The two most common MS-based methods for protein identification are peptide mass fingerprinting (PMF) and tandem MS (MS/MS).

PMF involves the use of chemical or enzymatic agents to digest proteins according to amino acid sequence cleavage specificity. The result of this controlled and sequence-specific cleavage is the production of a set of peptide fragments unique to each protein that represents a "fingerprint." The extent to which this fingerprint is unique to a given protein determines the ability to identify a given protein from the proteome confidently and uniquely. A caveat to identification by PMF is that the observed masses must be known to originate from a single (or small subset) of proteins; therefore, the presence of modifications or other proteins can be problematic.

The second approach used for protein identification is based on the information derived from the mass of a peptide augmented by the additional, sequence-related dissociation of the peptide. In MS/MS, first an ionized peptide peak is selected from the mixture of ions produced in the ion source of the MS instrument. The selected

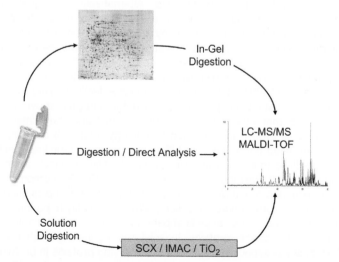

Fig. 2. Sample preparative workflows for MS-based proteomic biomarker discovery.

peptide molecular ion is fragmented, most commonly through activation by collisions with an inert gas (eg, collision-induced dissociation) into smaller-fragment ions carrying sequence information, which then are mass analyzed in a second scan event (ie, MS/MS). Peptides can be identified using various computational algorithms that match the observed tandem mass spectrum to a database of theoretical tandem mass spectra derived from known peptide sequences (reviewed in Ref. 1). This approach greatly reduces the number of peptides needed for protein identification with conventional instrumentation. Although this method results in the identification of peptides in the strictest sense, there are an abundance of bioinformatic algorithms to query and match the sequence of an identified peptide to the protein from which it was liberated from in silico translated genomic sequences.[1]

Difference gel electrophoresis (DIGE) is a modification of 2D-PAGE that requires only a single gel to detect differences between two protein samples reproducibly.[2] DIGE circumvents the reproducibility problems associated with comparing two different 2D gels. The principle of the method is simple: two different protein mixtures are labeled with two different fluorophores, 1-(5-carboxypentyl)-1'-propylindocarbo-cyanine halide (Cy3) N-hydroxysuccinimidyl ester and 1-(5-carboxypentyl)-1'-methyl-indodi-carbocyanine halide (Cy5) N-hydroxysuccinimidyl ester fluorescent dyes, respectively. The labeled proteins are mixed and resolved in the same 2D gel, thus making it possible to run two different samples in the same gel (see **Fig. 1**). Protein spots are detected by fluorescence imaging immediately after electrophoresis using a dual-laser scanning device with different excitation/emission filters to generate two separate images. The images are compared computationally, fluorescent signals are normalized, and spot volumes are quantified. Proteins whose abundances are found differ in the two samples can be excised from the gel, digested, and analyzed by MS for peptide/protein identification.

Although it is a robust format, there has been a significant shift from 2D-PAGE–based techniques toward capillary liquid chromatography (LC)-based methods to conduct proteomic investigations because of a number of well-recognized drawbacks related to the incompatibility of certain proteins with 2D-PAGE or the limits of sensitivity afforded by the dyes used for protein visualization.[3,4] Furthermore, a gel format is difficult to integrate online with MS analysis, thus limiting its use for broad proteome coverage and high-throughput proteomics. Alternatively, "shotgun" proteomic approaches have been developed in which a chemically or enzymatically digested proteomic sample is resolved in-solution by LC that can be conducted offline or coupled directly online by electrospray ionization to sequence-based protein identification by MS/MS.[3,4] The ability of capillary-based separations coupled directly online with MS to provide broad proteome coverage was demonstrated initially by the identification of more than 1000 proteins in a single analysis, facilitating higher-throughput proteomic analyses that have higher protein coverage and greater overall sensitivity than 2D-PAGE MS methods.[5] Both single-dimensional and multidimensional (eg, the multidimensional protein identification technology [MudPIT]) capillary LC techniques have been used online with MS/MS in numerous proteomics investigations, and now hundreds to thousands of proteins are identified routinely in an analysis. By increasing sensitivity beyond that possible with 2D-PAGE, proteomic measurements can be extended to smaller cell populations or tissue samples such as those obtained from laser-capture microdissection (LCM).[6] The ability to perform proteomic experiments with high dynamic range is of paramount importance, enabling the identification of low-abundance proteins in mixtures containing higher-abundance proteins. This ability is especially important in identifying proteins in biofluids, where the dynamic range of protein concentration is likely to span more than 10 logs.[7]

QUANTITATIVE PROTEOMICS

Although the broad proteomic identification capabilities of these solution-based techniques combined with MS are powerful, the goal ultimate of proteomics is not simply to provide a protein catalog but to enable the annotation of changes in protein abundance commensurate with cellular perturbation or activation. Label-free quantitation (often termed "spectral counting") is growing in popularity in the proteomics community and relies on the premise that increased numbers of peptide identifications per protein reflect the overall abundance of that protein in a given sample.[8] Nonetheless, accurate and precise measurement of relative peptide abundance probably is achievable only by using stable-isotope labeling strategies. Quantitative MS has a long history in small-molecule analyses in drug metabolism and pharmacokinetic studies, where surrogate standards are synthesized with stable isotope atoms and used in the LC-MS/MS workflow. The comparison of the endogenous species against these standards can provide a relative measure of abundance.[9] Application of this concept to protein MS includes metabolic labeling in which stable isotopes are incorporated into proteins in cell culture systems during translation or after proteome isolation using protein-reactive tags that possess isotope "codes."

^{15}N-Labeling

^{15}N-labeling is based on the growth of one population of cells in a culture medium containing the natural abundance of nitrogen isotopes and another in culture medium enriched in the stable "heavy" isotope, ^{15}N.[10] The two populations of cells are harvested and pooled. After protein extraction and digestion, the peptides are analyzed by LC-MS/MS.[11] Through analysis by MS, the two separate pools of proteins can be distinguished on the basis of the isotope pattern, because one set of peptides contains the natural abundance of nitrogen isotopes, but proteins from the other set are enriched in ^{15}N. This enrichment effectively "increases" the mass of ^{15}N-labeled peptides as compared with their unlabeled counterparts. The resulting mass spectra contain paired peaks of peptides. A relative quantitative measure of the abundance of the peptides can be extracted from the ratio of the isotope pairs (isotopomers), and inferences can be made regarding the relative abundance of the proteins from which the peptides originated. Therefore, MS analysis is used to compare the relative amounts of each protein in the two different samples and also to identify the protein. Importantly, the tandem mass spectra of ^{14}N- and ^{15}N-labeled peptides are qualitatively similar.

Stable-Isotope Labeling by Amino Acids in Cell Culture

Stable-isotope labeling by amino acids in cell culture (SILAC) has been used successfully to study quantitative changes in protein synthesis and degradation, protein–protein interactions, and specific posttranslational protein modifications, among other applications.[12] When SILAC is used to conduct proteome-scale relative quantitation, one cell population is cultured in normal cell culture medium and another population is cultured in medium supplemented with either a single amino acid or multiple amino acids that possess stable heavy-isotope atoms (^{13}C, ^{2}H, ^{15}N, or ^{18}O).[12] Cells grown in the medium supplemented with heavy-isotope amino acids incorporate these atoms into protein translation, producing proteins identical to those from cells grown in normal medium in all respects except for their greater mass resulting from the number of heavy amino acids in the sequence. Both light- and heavy-labeled cell populations are grown for at least six passages in the SILAC medium. The most significant limitation of this technique pertains to the adaptation of individual cell cultures to dialyzed serum, which may alter the biologic behavior of cell lines. The use of dialyzed serum in the culture medium is necessary to avoid the contribution of natural stable-isotope abundance amino acids in the serum of the heavy-labeled cell culture.

Isotope-Coded Affinity Tags/Isobaric Tag for Relative and Absolute Quantitation

The labeling strategies that use isotopically defined media offer the greatest precision and the broadest proteome coverage. As mentioned previously, however, metabolic labeling is limited to cells that can be cultured in special medium. Postextraction isotopic labeling is universally applicable to proteins extracted from every conceivable source. Postextraction labeling also makes possible the use of a less complex mixture in some schemes and can aid identification by providing an additional sequence constraint. Postextraction isotopic labeling, however, does require additional sample processing, necessarily results in decreased protein coverage, and possibly decreases quantitative precision and/or accuracy.

The most popular postextraction methodology uses a pair of isotope-coded affinity tags (ICAT) that allow global measurements of the relative abundances of peptides from virtually any source.[13] ICAT reagents can be thought of as possessing three vital chemical moieties: an iodoacetyl functionality that is used to modify covalently the sulfhydryls of reduced cysteinyl residues, an ethylene glycol linker region that can be synthesized to possess either eight protons (d_0) or eight deuterons (d_8), and a biotin moiety that allows the selective isolation of ICAT-labeled peptides by avidin-affinity chromatography. In ICAT labeling, the two cell extracts to be compared are each labeled with either the d_0 or the d_8 version of ICAT, combined and digested, and the ICAT-labeled peptides are isolated by avidin-affinity chromatography. Hence, ICAT labeling results in differentially stable-isotope–labeled "sister" cysteinyl-containing polypeptides whose masses are separated by exactly the mass of the heavy ICAT label, or approximately 8 Da.

Similar in methodology to the ICAT reagent, the isobaric tag for relative and absolute quantitation (iTRAQ, Applied Biosystems, Inc.) reagents can be used to label peptide mixtures for quantitation but with some distinct, and arguably improved, differences.[14] The iTRAQ reagents are designed similarly to the ICAT reagents but are amine specific, rather than cysteine-specific like the ICAT reagents. Therefore, in theory, all peptides from a digested lysate can be analyzed by MS, and there is no need for affinity chromatography. In addition, up to eight different sample types can be labeled for comparison, allowing greater flexibility in experimental design. The iTRAQ methodology, however, relies on the fragmentation of the attached reagent during MS/MS, releasing reporter ions observed at very low mass (m/z 113-119, 121) that are necessary for quantitation. Inherently different from the traditional MS/MS analyses with the ICAT reagent (identified and quantitated as a fixed modification on all peptides), iTRAQ is directly applicable to some MS platforms (eg, matrix-assisted laser desorption/ionization–time of flight/time of flight [MALDI TOF/TOF]) but requires modified instrumental parameters in others (eg, ion trap MS) to isolate and observe the reporter ions during MS/MS.

POSTTRANSLATIONAL MODIFICATIONS: PHOSPHORYLATION

One of the key factors affecting protein function is the presence of posttranslation modifications (PTMs). A plethora of known (and probably many more as yet unknown) modifications affect protein function; among them are acetylation, methylation, sulfation, and glycosylation. One of the most important PTMs used to modulate protein activity and propagate signals within cellular pathways and networks is reversible phosphorylation.[15] Cellular processes ranging from cell-cycle progression, differentiation, development, peptide hormone response, and adaptation are all regulated by protein phosphorylation. Although effective methods of identifying and determining relative protein abundances have been developed, the delineation of the function of a protein solely from changes in abundance changes provides only a limited view of the proteome, because numerous vital activities of proteins are modulated by phosphorylation.

The predominant means of determining protein phosphorylation relies on the use of high-affinity reagents such as anti-phosphoamino acid–specific monoclonal antibodies. Although these affinity-based detection methods can determine whether a protein is phosphorylated, they may not identify the specific site of modification, information that is important because an identical modification at a different site within the same protein can have a very different effect on the activity of a protein. In addition, several different enzymes may modify a single protein, each indicating an active cell pathway. Although MS measurements can confirm the presence of a phosphate group on a peptide, MS/MS is necessary to establish the specific site of phosphorylation. In the case of phosphopeptides, however, the phosphate group usually dissociates from the phosphorylated residue during traditional collision-induced dissociation peptide fragmentation, preventing identification of the site of the phosphate modification. A relatively new technology, electron transfer dissociation, uses a different peptide fragmentation process in which the posttranslational modification remains attached to the residue during MS/MS, permitting the precise site of phosphorylation to be determined.[16] Used separately or in tandem, these MS technologies make it possible to distinguish these modifications specifically, allowing a better understanding of the biologic processes involved.

One of the major difficulties in the analysis of phosphopeptides is their relatively low-abundance relative to other peptides in the sample. A common method of enriching a sample for phosphopeptides before MS analysis is the use of antibodies to immunoprecipitate a phosphorylated protein(s) from a mixture or to select phosphopeptides from a mixture containing all types of modified and unmodified peptides. In addition, phosphopeptide-specific antibodies can be coupled covalently to a solid support and packed within a chromatography column. A complex mixture of peptides then is passed over the column. The antibody captures the phosphopeptides, and the rest of the peptides pass directly through. This approach has been used to monitor changes in the phosphorylation states of proteins extracted from murine fibroblast L929 cells treated with tumor necrosis factor-α.[17] In this study, proteins were extracted from L929 cells at various time-points, were separated by 2D-PAGE, and were electroblotted onto a polyvinylidene fluoride membrane or silver stained. The blot was immunostained using an anti-pTyr monoclonal antibody to enable the identification of the proteins and to quantify any changes in the phosphorylation state-of-the proteins over time. The protein spots that immunostained with the anti-pTyr antibody were correlated with their position on the silver-stained gel. These gel spots were excised from the 2D-PAGE gel, digested with trypsin, and analyzed by MALDI TOF MS to identify the phosphoprotein. Twenty-one different phosphoproteins were identified within the L929 cell lysates, including eight that showed a time-dependent change in the phosphorylation state.

More recently, several affinity-based methods of extracting phosphoproteins or phosphopeptides from complex mixtures have been developed (see **Fig. 2**). The first of these is immobilized metal affinity chromatography (IMAC).[18] In IMAC, trivalent cations such as Fe^{3+} or Ga^{3+} are bound to a solid support. Passing a complex mixture over the column results in an enrichment of the phosphorylated species because of the affinity of the phosphate moiety for the metal ion. After the column is washed, the remaining bound species are eluted using high-pH or phosphate buffer. The eluted peptides can be analyzed using LC-MS to identify the phosphorylated peptide. An alternate and promising new methodology for phosphopeptide enrichment relies on the affinity of titanium dioxide (TiO$_2$) for phosphate groups. This method has been used successfully in complex mixtures to enrich low-abundance phosphopeptides selectively.[19]

Several groups recently have performed a number of phosphoproteome analyses demonstrating the effectiveness of these enrichment techniques and the improved coverage they afford. Dephoure and colleagues[20] describe experiments in HeLa cells to characterize protein phosphorylation at different stages of the cell cycle using isotope labeling and multiple fractionation (strong cation exchange, SCX) and enrichment (IMAC/TiO$_2$) to maximize recovery and identification. More than 14,000 sites of phosphorylation were identified in the analysis, and more than 1000 were increased in phosphorylation during mitosis. Olsen and colleagues[21] used a three-way isotope labeling in HeLa cells and a similar SCX-TiO$_2$ methodology to identify more than 2200 proteins with 6600 phosphorylation sites after different treatments with epidermal growth factor.

CLINICAL PROTEOMICS: APPLICATIONS TO CANCER
Cell Culture

Early detection of cancer is critical for better prognosis and positive outcome. To this end, reliable biomarkers of cancer are increasingly sought. The discovery of cancer-specific biomarkers from biofluids such as plasma and urine has proven challenging, in part because of the typically low-abundance of these markers in a background of highly diverse proteins with a broad dynamic range. Cell culture–based cancer model systems are used not only as a potential abundant source of cancer-specific markers but also as a means to understand better the molecular basis of this complex disease. This strategy allows experimental control for the measurement of biochemical cellular end points.

Currently an aggressive effort is being made to identify cancer biomarkers using proteomics and MS-based technologies in cell culture. Thus far most studies have focused on the identification of cancer biomarkers, partly because of the commercial availability of immortalized cancer cell lines. Bladder cancer is the fourth most common cancer in the United States, and its prognosis depends heavily on whether the tumor becomes invasive. Recently, using 2D LC-MS/MS, chemokine (C-X-C motif) ligand 1 (CXCL-1) has been identified as a potential novel biomarker in six bladder cell lines.[22] Novel proteins regulated by matrix metalloproteinases in a human prostate cell line have been identified by a label-free quantitative approach.[23] Sardana and colleagues[24] characterized conditioned medium from three human prostate cancer cell lines (PC3 [bone metastasis], LNCaP [lymph node metastasis], and 22Rv1 [localized to prostate]) to identify secreted proteins that could serve as novel prostate cancer biomarkers. Four candidates were found (follistatin, chemokine [C-X-C motif] ligand 16, pentraxin 3, and spondin 2) and were validated further in human sera from patients with or without prostate cancer. Similarly, three conditioned breast cancer cell lines (MCF-10A, BT474, and MDA-MB-468) were used to identify potential markers secreted in the culture medium.[25] Three kallikreins (KLK5, KLK6, and KLK10) and the protease inhibitor elafin were identified from BT474 and MDA-MB-468 in the cell-free medium and were validated further by their presence in various biologic samples.[25] An alternative approach using a 2D-PAGE and MALDI TOF MS analysis of a colorectal cancer secretome was applied successfully in the identification of collapsin response mediator protein-2, a protein that is present in early stage tumors and lymph node metastatic foci.[26] A novel targeted approach using human prostate and bladder stromal cells resulted in the identification of several glycoproteins, including cathepsin L, follistatin-related protein, neuroendocrine convertase 2, and tumor necrosis factor receptor superfamily member 11B, as potential markers involved in signaling and differentiation.[27] The use of cell culture models allows the discovery of cancer biomarkers and also can be used to identify therapeutic targets. For example, two recent studies have investigated response to treatment using MS-based proteomics. Serotonin receptors were identified as potential targets of sulforaphane (increasingly recognized as a potential chemopreventative agent present in high levels in cruciferous vegetables) in Caco-2 cells, a model of colon cancer.[28] Results from other investigations have implicated heat-shock protein 27 as a potential biomarker for monitoring resistance to chemotherapy in pancreatic cancer cells.[29]

A recent study by Yang and colleagues[30] using a gel-based MS approach identified more than 150 unique proteins from a cell supernatant fraction collected from cells carrying the HCV genotype 2a. Fatty acid synthase (FASN) was highly enriched, and on further investigation the investigators found that blocking FASN activity by inhibitors or RNA interference decreased HCV production and suppressed viral replication, respectively. In addition, the study found that FASN is required for the expression of claudin-1, a protein that has been suggested to be a co-receptor for the entry of HCV into cells. In another study using HaCaT cells, a model of proliferating keratinocytes, proteomics was used to identify a novel biomarker, CD98, which is increased in abundance in basal amplifying keratinocytes.[31]

TISSUE-BASED MASS SPECTROMETRY
Fresh-Frozen Tissues

Fresh-frozen tissues are arguably the preferred tissue source for proteomic analyses, although this paradigm is beginning to shift, as discussed later in this article. These samples often are deemed quite precious and are difficult to gather in significant quantities and cohorts. Nonetheless, several successful cancer biomarker investigations have been performed using fresh-frozen tissues. A recent effort investigated differences between freshly collected breast cancer and normal tissues. The primary workflow employed a two-pronged approach in which total cell lysates were resolved by 1D PAGE along with a strategy for membrane protein enrichment of pooled and matched metastatic (node-positive) and nonmetastatic (node-negative) cancer tissues before MS analysis. Label-free quantitation of more than 1000 proteins resulted in the identification of numerous proteins that were more abundant in breast cancer as than in normal healthy breast tissue.[32] Proteins implicated in breast cancer such as L-plastin and STAT1, as well as a variety of signal transduction proteins including IQGAP1 (which binds to activated CDC42 GAP) and Rab-like GTPase, were identified at increased abundance levels in breast cancer tissue. Several proteins, including lactadherin (which promotes cancer cell adhesion), were found to be differentially abundant in metastatic and nonmetastatic breast cancer tissue. Multiple proteins were further verified using Western blot analysis and immunohistochemistry.

In another study, LCM was used to collect cells from brain microvascular endothelium using an immuno-based staining technique to target various cell types of interest.[33] Cellular lysates from approximately 5000 cells immunostained with anti-CD31 were separated by 1D-PAGE followed by in-gel digestion of multiple fractions and analysis by LC-MS/MS. Nearly 900 proteins were identified in the study; 20% were identified by multiple unique peptides. Of interest in the analysis was the identification of multiple blood–brain barrier–related proteins that were expected to be enriched (a finding that corroborates previously reported results) and several proteins such as myelin basic protein and glial acidic fibrillary protein, thought to be expressed or localized in oligodendrocytes and astrocytes/neurons, respectively—that were not expected to be associated with brain microvascular endothelium. The ability to identify such a significant number of proteins from a minimal and cell-type–specific sample holds tremendous promise for directed tissue-based MS investigations of the tumor microenvironment.

Formalin-Fixed Paraffin-Embedded Tissues

To correlate the biomarker–tumor connection, tumor biopsies must be performed, and other biochemical methods, such as immunohistochemistry (IHC), or imaging methods must be used to validate the site of origination of a given protein biomarker. The extraction of tumor material, either surgically or through a needle biopsy, is highly invasive, however, and the cost (in both time and money) of obtaining sizable cohorts of samples makes such studies almost impractical for discovery-driven biomarker research. There is an immense archive of tumors in the form of formalin-fixed paraffin-embedded (FFPE) tissues that, although routinely used for IHC in situ hybridization studies, have been underutilized in MS-based proteomics, in large part because of the notion that formaldehyde-induced inter- and intramolecular covalent cross-links render proteins intractable to traditional techniques of proteomic sample preparation for high-throughput MS analysis. Because a substantial portion of the structure of a given protein is solvent inaccessible, it is conceivable that the majority of the primary sequence may be protected from formaldehyde modification. Enzymatic digestion probably will produce an ensemble of peptides that are readily identifiable by MS.

The initial and groundbreaking proteomic study from FFPE tissue combined the use of LCM with MS in the investigation of prostate cancer and benign prostatic hyperplasia, using cells captured from the same archived prostate thin-tissue section.[34] Several hundred proteins were identified from these LCM samples, including a variety of prostate-related proteins such as prostatic acid phosphatase and prostate-specific antigen. This analysis also resulted in the identification of proteins distinct to each pathology, such as growth differentiation factor 15, which was identified solely from the prostate cancer cells. A significant finding emerging from this investigation was the comparative recovery of peptides from FFPE tissue and fresh-frozen tissue, suggesting that archival FFPE tissues are a valuable new clinical sample source for the MS-based discovery of cancer biomarkers.

More recently, Hwang and colleagues[35] developed a direct tissue proteomics methodology that interrogates the proteomes of these samples and also has the ability to determine the relative quantitation of proteins using isotope-dilution MS techniques (as discussed later) and using IHC to confirm the results. Patel and colleagues[36] performed a retrospective analysis of cancer differentiation in multiple FFPE tissues of head and neck squamous cell carcinoma. From hundreds of protein identifications within each subset, particular differentially abundant proteins that were identified by LC-MS/MS were validated against a larger tissue microarray sample set. Among these proteins were cytokeratin 4 and desmoplakin, both of which have been described previously as being altered in response to cellular differentiation. Another study evaluated the proteome of precursor pancreatic cancer lesions, identifying deleted in malignant brain tumors-1 and tissue transglutaminase, both of which were verified by IHC in multiple microarray sections of intraductal papillary mucinous neoplasm (IPMN) tissue as having increased abundance in distinct regions of the IPMN epithelium and/or in the juxta-tumoral stroma, but not in non-neoplastic pancreas.[37] The ability to access archival tumor tissues for proteomic research makes it possible to quantify differentially abundant proteins from the tumor microenvironment across hundreds of samples.

Tissue Imaging

A novel application of MALDI for direct mass spectral imaging of thin sections of tissue was reported more than a decade ago and is drawing increasing attention as a technique for identifying biomarkers from tissue.[38] Direct tissue imaging by MALDI is enabled by the ability to lay a thin coat of the energy-absorbing MALDI matrix solution directly onto the surface of tissue sections. When impinged by a nitrogen laser, the energy imparted to the matrix is transferred to the co-crystallized substrate, in this case biochemicals and macromolecules in the tissue section, followed by their desorption and ionization. The actual image is reconstructed after rastering the tissue section with the laser and is based on the mass spectral profile composite (or a selected m/z subset) of the detected biochemicals and macromolecules and the location within a Cartesian coordinate on the tissue where the laser was directed. The resolution of the resulting image is constrained primarily by the focal diameter of the laser beam, typically on the order of 100 to 150 μm. Although this resolution is significantly less than the average 10-μm human cell, it has provided compelling images of tissue sections with good definition of structures based on the detection of specific molecular species. Direct tissue imaging by MALDI can provide detailed information regarding the localization of specific molecules in an unbiased fashion.

Lemaire and colleagues[39] recently used MALDI imaging to identify biomarkers for the detection of ovarian carcinoma. In this investigation, 25 specimens of ovarian carcinoma and 23 benign ovarian tissue specimens were collected from women undergoing ovarian tumor resection. Thin sections (10–12 μm) were cut with a cryostat, thaw-mounted on MALDI target plates, and analyzed by MALDI TOF MS. Approximately 100 individual peptide peaks were observable per tissue section from m/z 500 to 20,000. A comparative bioinformatic analysis of the spectra revealed a peak at m/z 9744 that was prevalent in 80% of the ovarian carcinoma samples and was not evident in the benign tumors. The investigators purified and identified this peptide by extracting the tissues with HCl and fractionating the extract by C18 reversed-phase LC. Analysis of each of the LC fractions by MALDI TOF enabled the fraction containing the peptide at m/z 9744 to be identified. This fraction was digested with trypsin and analyzed by MALDI TOF for PMF and by nanoESI qTOF for MS/MS-based sequence analysis. This analysis identified peptides corresponding to 70% sequence coverage of Reg-alpha, a protein involved in the 11S proteasome activator complex. An alignment of the identified peptides suggested that this 9743-Da peptide peak is a C-terminal fragment of the 28-kDa Reg-alpha holoprotein. These investigators developed an antibody to the C-terminal region of Reg-alpha that was used for validation by Western blot and immunocytochemistry analyses, which demonstrated that Reg-alpha was present in 88.8% of the carcinoma specimens and 18.7% of the benign tumor specimens.

Another novel application of MALDI-based tissue imaging was published by Chaurand and colleagues,[40] who used this technology to monitor the evolution of protein expression throughout prostate development in a mouse model. In this study, prostates from CD-1 transgenic mice (bearing the large-T antigen) were analyzed by imaging MS and were compared with prostates from CD-1 normal mice along a defined developmental time-course from week 1 through 40. Cells in the prostates of these large-T antigen–bearing mice are known to continue proliferating actively well after the normal halt of proliferation at week 5 and to develop prostate cancer at a penetrance of 100%. The goal of the study was to identify proteins associated with normal prostate development and prostate cancer tumorigenesis. This investigation identified two soluble and secreted proteins, probasin and spermine-binding protein, in mature prostates, both of which were absent in the tumors of the large-T antigen–transgenic mice. An interesting result of this investigation was identification of cyclophilin A, which was detected as modified with an α-N-terminal acetylation in both normal and tumor-bearing prostates, although it was not possible to discern which cells within the prostate were responsible for expression of this protein.

BIOFLUID PROTEOMICS
Serum/Plasma

Because blood continuously perfuses all tissues of the body, including sites of emerging tumors, this constant biochemical flux is likely to result in the release and/or active secretion of protein species into the peripheral circulation, resulting in a rich biologic milieu for potential discovery and assay of tumor markers. These complex serum proteomic patterns and multi-analyte profiles are thought to contain biologic information regarding the molecular etiology of tumorigenesis and tumor progression and therefore can be evaluated for diagnostic features that can be used to identify and characterize all the categories or tumor markers described in earlier sections. This potentially rich spectrum of biomarkers, reflecting complex tumor–host cell interactions, sampled in serum, provides biologically complementary information that, when used together in panels, could provide greater diagnostic accuracy than achieved with traditional single tumor markers. Despite this potential, a comprehensive characterization of the circulatory proteome is impossible with current technology because of the extreme dynamic range of protein concentrations, from the abundant proteins such as albumin (mg/mL) to the sought-after biomarkers that are hypothesized to be at much lower abundance (in levels of less than pg/mL).[7] Despite these challenges, much has been learned about the nature of this complex proteome, and many provocative results have stemmed from MS-based investigations of serum. Many of the early proteomic investigations into serum were aimed at developing improved analytic and technological capabilities, essentially efforts to increase the overall analytic dynamic range of identified proteins to that afforded by the typical two to three orders of magnitude that constrain most routine measurements possible by MS. Many of these efforts focused on devising clever methods of depletion, enrichment, separation, and pre-fractionation of serum proteins before MS analysis to decrease the overall dynamic range of protein concentration in the resulting sample and to increase the breadth and depth of the proteins identified in the MS experiment.

One of the first studies aimed at the broad identification of proteins in plasma incorporated 2D-PAGE with MS identification of the visualized protein spots. The strategy employed a workflow involving immunodepletion of nine of the most abundant serum proteins (albumin, haptoglobin, transferrin, transthyretin, α-1-antitrypsin, α-1-acid glycoprotein, hemopexin, and α-2-macroglobulin) followed by an extensive chromatographic fractionation by sequential anion-exchange and size-exclusion chromatography, resulting in a total of 74 plasma protein fractions, each of which was resolved by 2D-PAGE.[41] The resolved proteins visualized with Coomassie staining resulted in approximately 20,000 spots across all 74 gels. After accounting for redundant spots, approximately 3700 unique protein spots were excised from the gels, digested with trypsin, and analyzed by MS. This analysis identified 1800 of the resolved proteins that corresponded to 350 unique proteins. Although this investigation represented the broadest annotation of the plasma proteome at the time, the strategy used suffered from the laborious nature of the workflow that renders large case-control studies unfeasible.

Although not reviewed extensively here (see Ref. 42 for a recent review), an interesting feature of many investigations that have employed surface-enhanced laser desorption/ionization (SELDI) TOF MS has been the consistent observation that m/z values of low molecular weight (LMW) consistently possess the key information for distinguishing samples in case-control studies. These key m/z values typically are less than 15 kDa, suggesting that the LMW serum proteome may provide useful biomarkers for the early detection of cancer. Indeed, LMW human serum proteins, peptides, and other small components have been associated with pathologies such as cancer, diabetes, and cardiovascular and infectious diseases. A simple method for enriching the LMW components in serum has been developed and used in conjunction with multidimensional chromatographic fractionation and MS analysis to identify the constituents in this LMW compartment.[43] The methodology employs dilution of serum with acetonitrile, which acts to disrupt protein–protein interactions, followed by a simple centrifugal ultrafiltration. This workflow was developed based on the hypothesis that LMW peptides are likely to be bound to larger-mass, highly abundant proteins, which, if released, could be selectively "filtered" through a low molecular-weight-cutoff (MWCO) membrane. Indeed, analysis of the LMW serum proteome that was recovered through a 30-kDa MWCO filter resulted in the identification of 341 proteins, many of which possess molecular masses much greater than 30 kDa. It was concluded that the LMW serum proteome is comprised largely of proteolytic fragments.

This investigation resulted in the sobering realization that serum proteomic workflows that employ depletion may concomitantly be effectively removing LMW biomarkers that are noncovalently associated with the depleted proteins.[44] This notion led to a number of investigations that actually exploited this interaction to enrich selectively for those LMW peptides bound to high-mass, highly abundant serum proteins. The first study to investigate this hypothesis used a strategy in which antibodies against albumin, IgA, IgG, IgM, apolipoprotein, and transferrins were used to capture these proteins specifically, along with any associated peptides.[45] The LMW peptides were filtered through a 30-kDa MWCO filter, digested, and analyzed by LC-MS/MS, resulting in the identification of more than 200 proteins. The interesting finding from this study was that 12 of the proteins identified through this workflow are used currently as clinical biomarkers. This study was the first to show definite evidence that a potential archive of diagnostic information may be bound to large, highly abundant circulatory proteins that are not cleared rapidly by glomerular filtration. Lowenthal and colleagues[46] exploited this interaction in a biomarker investigation for ovarian cancer in which they pooled sera from a human disease study set (high-risk persons without cancer, n = 40; stage I ovarian cancer, n = 30; stage III ovarian cancer, n = 40). In their study, albumin was isolated by affinity capture, and the albumin-associated proteins and peptides were analyzed by LC-MS/MS. Their investigation identified 1208 proteins from the three pools of albumin-enriched serum. This investigation validated a number of proteolytic fragments of larger molecules that may be cancer related and were confirmed immunologically in blood by Western blotting and peptide immunocompetition. Among these, BRCA2, a 390-kDa low-abundance nuclear protein known to be associated with increased cancer susceptibility, was represented in sera as a series of specific fragments bound to albumin.

Despite the challenges associated with conducting proteomic investigations in serum, current efforts have had substantial success in identifying potential cancer biomarkers. A recent provocative study used a well-characterized genetically engineered mouse model of pancreatic cancer. In this investigation plasma was sampled from mice at early and advanced stages of pancreatic tumor development and from matched controls.[47] Using a proteomic approach based on extensive protein fractionation, this team identified 1442 proteins that were distributed across seven orders of magnitude of abundance in plasma. Although this result is impressive in its own right, the relevance of this study lay in the teams' ability to distill a panel of five proteins (LCN2, TIMP1, REG1A, REG3, and IGFBP4) that were increased in abundance in mouse serum at an early stage of tumor development. The abundance levels of these candidate markers were assessed in a blinded study of samples from 26 human patients in the Carotene and Retinol Efficacy Trial cohort. The results showed that the markers could be used to distinguish pancreatic cancer cases from matched controls in plasma obtained between 7 and 13 months before the development of symptoms and clinical diagnosis of pancreatic cancer.

Proximal Fluids

Although it is clear that, from an analytic perspective, the preferred sample for conducting protein biomarker discovery is tissue, in large part because of the estimated high local concentration of disease-specific proteins, the preferred clinical sample for patient screening and monitoring usually is serum. Although serum is the preferred clinical sample, the analytic challenges are great because of the overall dynamic range of protein concentration and the potential low concentration of biomarkers; particularly in early stage cancer. Proximal fluids are gaining increasing attention as a rich substrate for conducting biomarker discovery. The underlying hypothesis is that the fluids that are nearest the site of a malignancy are most likely to have a very high local concentration of soluble proteins and protein fragments that are produced as a result of active secretion and shedding from the tissue microenvironment. It is anticipated that the discovery of cancer-related biomarkers may be more facile from proximal fluids because of this high locoregional concentration of proteins that otherwise are greatly diluted in peripheral circulation. This concentration gradient is likely to span more than three orders of magnitude. For example, Sedlaczek and colleagues[48] recently reported a study that examined the average concentration of CA125 in serum, ascites, and cyst fluid in a population of 67 patients who had ovarian carcinoma. CA125, a protein biomarker, is measured clinically and used as a marker for follow-up of patients who have ovarian carcinoma. Although the level of abundance of CA125 in serum has been demonstrated to enable the detection of more than 80% of advanced ovarian carcinoma, this protein is much less useful for detecting early stage cancer. Nonetheless, CA125 is the most widely used biomarker for detecting ovarian cancer. If the serum level of CA125 is determined to be higher than 35 ng/mL, the patient is referred for more intensive clinical follow-up. Sedlaczek and colleagues found that the median level of abundance of CA125 from ascites and ovarian cyst fluid in patients who had serous carcinoma was 18,563 and 44,850 ng/mL, respectively, representing a concentration gradient greater than 1200-fold.

Cerebrospinal Fluid

Cerebrospinal fluid (CSF) is the fluid that bathes and protects the brain and spinal cord and has many putative functions. Although collecting CSF is more invasive (requiring lumbar puncture), the nature of its immediate environment makes it a rich resource for the detection and evaluation of many neurologic diseases and central nervous system afflictions. Although CSF has not been used widely in cancer biomarker investigations, multiple studies have used CSF to understand better Alzheimer's disease,[49] multiple sclerosis,[50] Creutzfeldt-Jakob disease,[51] and amyotrophic lateral sclerosis.[52] These studies have used a wide variety of sample preparation techniques including 1D- and 2D-PAGE, depletion, ultrafiltration, and fractionation, combined with multiple MS instrumentation such as SELDI, MALDI-TOF/TOF, and electrospray ionization (ESI) coupled to low- and high-resolution ion trap mass spectrometers.

Indeed, recent efforts at characterizing the global proteome of CSF have identified more than 2500 proteins with high confidence from three different experiments.[51] The first of these experimental methodologies used an initial fractionation of a pooled CSF sample by sodium dodecyl sulfate (SDS)-PAGE fractionation followed by in-gel digestion. These fractions were separated into two portions of 100 μg each, and each was further subjected to SCX chromatography, one using the MudPIT technology coupled online with MS and the other offline followed by MS analysis. The combined analyses identified 1474 proteins, showing good depth of coverage and identifying known CSF proteins. In the second study, more than 1500 proteins were identified from pre-fractionated CSF using acetonitrile precipitation to remove albumin and IgG, followed by labeling of the pre-fractions with the iTRAQ technology and analysis by MALDI-TOF/TOF MS.[51] Finally, a glycoproteomic analysis was performed using lectin affinity or hydrazide modification to identify 359 potential glycoproteins; approximately one fourth of these proteins had not been identified in the previous two studies. The results from these combined experiments show that multiple different MS platforms and workflows can be used in the analysis of this complex proximal fluid to evaluate differences in protein abundances in various disease states.[51]

To evaluate better the changes within CSF, a study evaluated the intra- and interindividual differences in CSF using depletion techniques and DIGE fractionation in combination with both MALDI- and ESI-based MS analyses.[49] Samples from six patients were taken twice with a 2-week interval between sample collection. Each sample pair was labeled with the appropriate dye along with a pooled standard (generated from all 12 samples) and evaluated by differential in-gel analysis. These experiments identified more than 1500 spots per gel, demonstrating the ability to reduce sample complexity and to track apparent changes in protein abundance (including proteins such as transthyretin and apolipoprotein E) within patients while also evaluating the significance of protein spots in common across all sample sets.

In another study patients who had Alzheimer's disease were treated with intravenous immunoglobulin, their CSF was collected at various times, and the response to treatment was monitored using the iTRAQ labeling technology.[53] Samples from two patients at four time-points were digested, labeled, and pooled, followed by strong cation-exchange fractionation of the pooled peptide mixtures and analysis by reversed-phase liquid chromatography (RPLC)-MALDI. Several hundred proteins were identified and quantified from more than 17,000 tandem mass spectra, including several proteins expected to change in response to the treatment such as hemopexin and α-2-macroglobulin. Additional visualization tools were developed, and Western blot analyses were performed to verify the results.[53] Although samples from only two patients were not statistically sufficient to generate broad claims, the analysis showed the ability to monitor relative changes in protein abundance both within and between patient samples. This study serves as another important example of the successful use of a protein/peptide-labeling technique in a biofluid, an endeavor that is notoriously difficult (certainly as applied to serum/plasma) while retaining sufficient complexity for deep annotation.

Nipple Aspirate

Several investigations have explored the utility of nipple aspirate fluid (NAF) in identifying biomarkers for the early detection of breast cancer.[54] Because the breast is comprised of a complex array of discrete ductal systems that begin at the nipple and branch throughout the breast toward the chest wall, it is hypothesized that protein biomarkers of breast cancer may be resident in the fluid that fills the lumen of these ducts. This fluid can be collected from the orifices that exit the nipple using noninvasive means (either by ductal lavage or nipple aspiration). In an early proof-of-principal demonstration of the ability to identify proteins from NAF using MS-based proteomics, 64 proteins were identified from NAF that was recovered from 90% of the subjects recruited to the study.[55] Although most of the identified proteins were proteins of moderate to high abundance, the abundance of 15 of these proteins reportedly is altered in the serum of patients who have breast cancer. The novel aspect of using NAF for breast cancer diagnosis is that the regional specificity of the sampling technique should provide an added level of confidence that observed differences in protein abundance arise from breast carcinoma.

Cervico-Vaginal Fluid

A novel biofluid in which biomarker discovery for diseases of the female pelvis and reproductive tract may be conducted is cervico-vaginal fluid (CVF), a combination of fluids that provide protection from vaginal infection. In an effort to characterize and understand better the protein complement of human CVF, Shaw and colleagues[56] used 1D-PAGE or SCX to identify 685 unique proteins from pooled samples. Samples were collected from multiple patients using gauze and were incubated further with phosphate-buffered saline for several hours before pooling and processing. Results from the combined experimental data were evaluated using pathway analysis software (Ingenuity) and gene ontology classifications to determine the biologic function and cellular localization of the proteins identified. Not surprisingly, given the nature of CVF, multiple defense-related proteins, proteolytic enzymes, and cytoskeletal and cell-adhesion proteins were identified. Specifically, multiple kallikreins, members of the serine protease family that are known to exist in human CVF, were identified by multiple peptides in the analysis and were evaluated further by ELISA, showing the ability to monitor protein abundances in this fluid.

Ascites Fluid

Ascites fluid is likely to contain an abundance of biochemical information related to the local tumor microenvironment, because it contains various cell types, including malignant cells and proteins that are shed from the tumor. Understanding the exact protein complement of these fluids may provide valuable insight into ovarian tumor growth and progression. In a study of four samples of ascites fluid from patients who had ovarian cancer, Gortzak-Uzan and colleagues[57] identified more than 2500 proteins using basic sample fractionation techniques, MudPIT technology, and gel-based MS analyses. These results were compared with reported proteomes of other related biofluids (plasma and urine), were evaluated further by comparison with multiple ovarian cancer microarray data sets, and select proteins of interest were measured by Western blot analysis. Using several bioinformatic applications to the data, the investigators suggested that 80 proteins that were observed in all four samples might be potential biomarkers; several novel targets were identified through the extensive post-MS analysis.

Novel Biofluid Sampling Techniques

Although progress has been made using traditional methods of sample acquisition and preparation, novel sampling techniques may offer interesting new opportunities for conducting biomarker discoveries from the loco-regional environment of disease, particularly in the case of cancer. A postoperative procedure for collecting tissue interstitial fluid (TIF) introduced by Celis and colleagues[58] harvests the biochemical "flotsam and jetsam" from the tumor microenvironment using samples of freshly resected tumor tissue. In the original demonstration of this procedure, Celis and colleagues[58] investigated the TIF proteome of breast carcinoma from 16 women who had primary operable high-risk grade 2 invasive breast cancer, none of whom had had previous surgery to the breast or received preoperative treatment. Tumor samples were obtained within 30 minutes of patient resection and were grossly cut into small pieces (1 mm^3), washed in 5 mL of phosphate-buffered saline (PBS), placed in a final volume of 0.8 mL of PBS, and incubated for 1 hour at 37°C in a humidified CO_2 incubator. The concentration of protein from the final TIF supernatant ranged remarkably, from 1 to 4 mg/mL. Each of the TIF supernatants was resolved by 2D-PAGE, and resolved proteins were analyzed by MALDI TOF MS to identify proteins. Although many highly abundant serum proteins, such as albumin, ferritin, a-1 antichymotrypsin, a-1 protease inhibitor, a-1 β glycoprotein, and haptoglobins 1 and 2, were evident, it was concluded that "the presence of multiple proteins in this fluid, as well as their multiple interactions, provides not only a rich source for discovering more specific diagnostic biomarkers, but also offers a model system to generate new therapeutic strategies to target the tumor microenvironment and to understand breast cancer progression."

Another novel collection methodology uses a strategy similar to fine-needle aspiration to access directly the tumor microenvironment secretome, the interstitial fluid immediately surrounding the tumor that is likely to contain shed and secreted proteins directly involved in tumor-host response. This capillary ultrafiltration sampling technique relies on a negative-pressure collection of sample using semipermeable membranes on the tip of a cannula that can be modified to target specifically the desired tumor or non–tumor cell microenvironments.[59] In situ application of this technique has been evaluated in a xenograft mouse model of fibrosarcoma and was able to identify differentially proteins known to be reflective of tumor progression and regression. Although more practical evaluation is needed, the technique of directed sample collection, with minimal invasiveness and while retaining tissue integrity, may provide the ability to investigate these interstitial fluids without adversely affecting the protein complement as a function of sampling.

In another interesting application of biofluid sampling, investigators have recovered fluids from induced blisters on the skin. In this technique, reducing vacuum pressures are applied to a suction chamber placed on the forearm until blisters form with sufficient fluid for collection by puncture.[60] Samples (and a serum standard of 30 pooled patient samples) were subjected to a variety of depletion methodologies and evaluated by 1D- and 2D-PAGE for biologic variation. Following digestion, peptides first were separated by offline SCX; then individual fractions were analyzed by RPLC-MS/MS. Under stringent criteria, approximately 400 proteins were identified in the analysis, nearly half of which were not identified in the standard serum sample analyzed similarly. From a subset of these blister fluid–specific proteins, several have been implicated as potential biomarkers for a wide range of diseases.

VALIDATION OF BIOMARKERS

Targeted analysis of protein expression typically is performed by Western blot analysis or by ELISA. Both these methods require one or more highly specific antibodies for each protein and are not capable of detecting more than a few proteins at a time. MS provides an alternative assay approach, relying on the discriminating power of mass analyzers to select a specific analyte and on ion current measurements for quantification.

Indeed, many small-molecule analytes (eg, drug metabolites and hormones) are measured routinely using this approach at high-throughput and with great precision (CVs < 5%).[61,62] In principle, this MS-based approach can provide absolute structural specificity for the selected molecule, and, in combination with appropriate stable isotope–labeled internal standards, can provide the concentration (eg, in terms of grams or moles) of the molecule present in the sample. In the typical application of this methodology, electrospray ionization is employed, followed by two stages of mass selection with a triple quadrupole MS: a first-stage (MS) selection of the mass of the intact analyte in the first quadrupole mass filter (the molecular ion) and, after fragmentation of the molecular ion by collision-induced dissociation in the collision quadrupole, a second stage of selection in the third quadrupole mass filter for specific transitions of the molecular ion, collectively generating a selected reaction-monitoring assay or, for plural reactions, a multiple reaction-monitoring (MRM) assay (**Fig. 3**). Operation of the MS instrument in this manner provides exquisite selectivity, because both the masses of the peptides and the specific masses of their fragment ions are monitored, and provides increased sensitivity because very narrow m/z regions are monitored during the analysis. A popular method for conducting quantitative measurements of a given protein by MRM is first to identify a tryptic peptide that ionizes well and is stable and reproducibly observable from the protein of interest. This peptide serves as the basis for synthesis of a stable-isotope standard (SIS) peptide to serve as an internal standard that is chemically identical to the native peptide but whose mass is greater according to the number of stable isotopes (eg, ^{13}C) present in the synthetic peptide mimic. Peptides suitable for use in MRM are selected based on several criteria, including size, ionization efficiency, the absence of cysteine and methionine residues, and their reproducible fragmentation to give several "fingerprint" fragment or transition ions resulting from collision-induced dissociation. In this methodology, known amounts of these SIS peptides are added to biologic samples, and after tryptic digestion the peptide digest is analyzed by LC-MS using a tandem mass spectrometer operating in MRM mode. The MS responses (eg, ion currents)

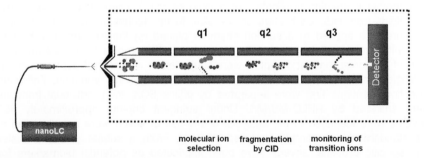

Fig. 3. Illustration of the operation of a triple quadrupole MS for conducting a selected reaction-monitoring/multiple reaction-monitoring assay.

of transition ions from the SIS and native peptides are integrated; the ratios of these responses provide a direct measure of the quantity of the native peptides because the amount of the SIS peptides initially spiked into the sample is known.

This specific methodology of using SIS peptides to conduct isotope-dilution MS was used first in 1996 by Barr and colleagues[63] to quantify apolipoprotein A-1 in a lyophilized serum reference material. This technology was extended to more complex matrix samples by Barnidge and colleagues[64] for quantification of rhodopsin from cell lysates. Gerber and colleagues[65] then demonstrated the utility of SDS-PAGE separation and in-gel digestion for sample enrichment and coined the term "AQUA" (for "absolute quantification") to denote the ability of this isotope-dilution technique to quantify peptide abundances relative to the SIS spiked into each sample. Although the term "AQUA" is gaining popularity, the quantification data obtained from this technique cannot be interpreted as providing absolute quantification of the protein in the original sample, given the losses that are inherent in any biochemical sample processing, including those associated with cellular lysis, protein denaturation, sample dilution/concentration, and incomplete digestion, to name a few. At best, this technique provides the ability to identify changes in the abundance of target peptides from an unlimited number of samples because of its ability to express all results as a ratio of a common SIS peptide. Care must be taken, however, in inferring changes in abundance of the intact protein in the original sample (eg, cell, tissue, or biofluid) based on the observed changes in peptide abundance from an MRM experiment.

The authors' laboratory has developed an MRM assay for quantification of asparagine synthetase (ASNS) from leukemic blasts.[66] Increases in ASNS abundance have been associated with the onset of resistance in acute lymphoblastic leukemia (ALL). Recent measurements using mRNA-based assays, however, have raised doubts about the importance of ASNS protein in the cellular mechanisms that confer drug resistance upon the leukemic cells.[67] The relationship between the mRNA levels for ASNS and intracellular protein concentrations in primary ALL was not established; the amount of ASNS mRNA was determined relative only to that from transcripts such as GAPDH.[67] Indeed, a recent study compared the correlation of asparaginase (ASNase) IC_{50} values against the relative abundance levels of ASNS mRNA and protein across a number of B- and T-cell–derived ALL cell lines that are known to have different expression levels of ASNS.[68] This study demonstrated that, although the level of ASNS mRNA does not correlate with ASNase sensitivity, the amount of ASNS protein correlates quite well.[68] Indeed, the authors concluded that "measurement of ASNS protein, rather than mRNA, may serve as a better indicator of ASNase sensitivity, potentially explaining the published inconsistencies between ASNS mRNA and drug sensitivity."[68] In the authors' MRM assay for ASNS, a SIS peptide of sequence ETF*EDSNLIPK (abbreviated "ETF*," where F* denotes a phenylalanine residue containing six ^{13}C atoms in the phenyl group) was synthesized and used to spike patient leukemic blast lysates. The ETFEDSNLIPK sequence corresponds to contiguous residues Glu-449 to Lys-459 in human ASNS.[69] In the present application, the complex peptide mixtures resulting from tryptic digestion of protein extracts were analyzed LC-MS/MS. After determination of the analytic figures of merit (eg, the lower limit of detection and quantification and the linear dynamic range), a series of measurements using this MRM assay were performed on protein extracts from blast cells in peripheral blood drawn from patients who had ALL. All four patients were multiply relapsed and previously had received ASNase as part of their therapy. The ETF peptide derived from ASNS was detected in the MRM assay in all four of the samples from patients who had ALL, allowing quantification of the amount of ASNS protein in the human leukemia cells (**Table 1**). These experiments are the first

Table 1 ASNS protein levels in samples from human leukemia patients			
Sample Identifier	ETFEDSNLIPK (amol)[a]	ASNS (amol)[b]	ASNS Molecules/Cell[c]
M082246	25 ± 8	50 ± 17	40 ± 10
M079837	170 ± 40	360 ± 80	200 ± 40
M080788	60 ± 20	130 ± 40	100 ± 30
M079880	30 ± 20	60 ± 40	100 ± 60

[a] Calculated by comparison to a known amount of the SIS peptide.
[b] Attomoles ASNS in 50 μg total cellular protein.
[c] Molecules per cell calculated based on initial leukemic blast cell count.

successful demonstration that concentrations of ASNS protein in human leukemia cells can be quantified using an MRM assay, illustrate the sensitivity and selectivity of MS-based methods for targeted detection of peptides in complex cellular mixtures, and open the way for clinical trials designed to probe the role of ASNS in chemotherapeutic resistance in ALL patient populations.

LOOKING AHEAD

As analytic technologies that comprise the central workflow for biomarker discovery using MS-based proteomic approaches develop and become more highly standardized, it is increasingly recognized that equivalent, if not greater, attention must be given to the standardization of sample collection and handling. Artifacts arising from nonspecific proteolysis and protein degradation are likely to be quite variable and to reflect not the underlying carcinogenesis but rather differences in pre-analytic factors such as sampling and handling. For example, a recent study demonstrating the ability to classify solid tumors based on the signature peptides produced by the action of exopeptidases postextraction[70] underscored the need for consistent sample handling before proteomic analysis. Even for samples such as FFPE tissues, the variability introduced by formalin-fixation time and length of storage are understood only poorly.[71] The variability introduced at every step in sample acquisition, storage, and processing have not been appraised in a systematic manner within a well-controlled study.

Although there are in vitro diagnostic applications that use MS (eg, the powerful assay used to screen newborns for inborn errors of metabolism),[61,62] there are many hurdles to overcome in translating MS technology to routine clinical assays of protein biomarkers from complex matrices. Perhaps in a more idealized workflow for translational biomarker development, high-affinity reagents would be generated against lead biomarkers forthcoming from MS-based discovery-driven investigations. These reagents, namely antibodies, which have a long and rigorously validated history of use in in vitro diagnostic applications, are likely to contribute significantly to the clinical adoption of newly discovered cancer biomarkers from MS-based proteomic investigations.

REFERENCES

1. McHugh L, Arthur JW. Computational methods for protein identification from mass spectrometry data. PLoS Comput Biol 2008;4(2):e1–e12.

2. Unlu M, Morgan ME, Minden JS. Difference gel electrophoresis: a single gel method for detecting changes in protein extracts. Electrophoresis 1997;18(11): 2071–7.
3. Domon B, Aebersold R. Mass spectrometry and protein analysis. Science 2006; 312(5771):212–7.
4. Aebersold R, Mann M. Mass spectrometry-based proteomics. Nature 2003; 422(6928):198–207.
5. Washburn MP, Wolters D, Yates JR. Large-scale analysis of the yeast proteome by multidimensional protein identification technology. Nat Biotechnol 2001;19(3): 242–7.
6. Bichsel VE, Liotta LA, Petricoin EF 3rd. Cancer proteomics: from biomarker discovery to signal pathway profiling. Cancer J 2001;7(1):69–78.
7. Anderson NL, Anderson NG. The human plasma proteome: history, character, and diagnostic prospects. Mol Cell Proteomics 2002;1(11):845–67.
8. Liu H, Sadygov RG, Yates JR 3rd. A model for random sampling and estimation of relative protein abundance in shotgun proteomics. Anal Chem 2004;76(14): 4193–201.
9. De Leenheer AP, Lefevere MF, Lambert WE, et al. Isotope-dilution mass spectrometry in clinical chemistry. Adv Clin Chem 1985;24:111–61.
10. Oda Y, Huang K, Cross FR, et al. Accurate quantitation of protein expression and site-specific phosphorylation. Proc Natl Acad Sci USA 1999;96(12):6591–6.
11. Conrads TP, Alving K, Veemstra TD, et al. Quantitative analysis of bacterial and mammalian proteomes using a combination of cysteine affinity tags and 15N-metabolic labeling. Anal Chem 2001;73(9):2132–9.
12. Ong SE, Blagoev B, Kratchmarova I, et al. Stable isotope labeling by amino acids in cell culture, SILAC, as a simple and accurate approach to expression proteomics. Mol Cell Proteomics 2002;1(5):376–86.
13. Gygi SP, Rist B, Gerber SA, et al. Quantitative analysis of complex protein mixtures using isotope-coded affinity tags. Nat Biotechnol 1999;17(10):994–9.
14. Chong PK, Gan CS, Pham TK, et al. Isobaric tags for relative and absolute quantitation (iTRAQ) reproducibility: implication of multiple injections. J Proteome Res 2006;5(5):1232–40.
15. Cohen P. The regulation of protein function by multisite phosphorylation—a 25 year update. Trends Biochem Sci 2000;25(12):596–601.
16. Coon JJ, Ueberheide B, Syka JE, et al. Protein identification using sequential ion/ion reactions and tandem mass spectrometry. Proc Natl Acad Sci USA 2005; 102(27):9463–8.
17. Yanagida M, Miura Y, Yagasaki K, et al. Matrix assisted laser desorption/ionization-time of flight-mass spectrometry analysis of proteins detected by anti-phosphotyrosine antibody on two-dimensional-gels of fibroblast cell lysates after tumor necrosis factor-alpha stimulation. Electrophoresis 2000;21(9):1890–8.
18. Neville DC, Rozanas CR, Price EM, et al. Evidence for phosphorylation of serine 753 in CFTR using a novel metal-ion affinity resin and matrix-assisted laser desorption mass spectrometry. Protein Sci 1997;6(11):2436–45.
19. Pinkse MW, Uitto PM, Hilhorst MJ, et al. Selective isolation at the femtomole level of phosphopeptides from proteolytic digests using 2D-NanoLC-ESI-MS/MS and titanium oxide precolumns. Anal Chem 2004;76(14):3935–43.
20. Dephoure N, Zhou C, Villen J, et al. A quantitative atlas of mitotic phosphorylation. Proc Natl Acad Sci USA 2008;105(31):10762–7.
21. Olsen JV, Blagoev B, Gnad F, et al. Global, in vivo, and site-specific phosphorylation dynamics in signaling networks. Cell 2006;127(3):635–48.

22. Kawanishi H, Matsui Y, Ito M, et al. Secreted CXCL1 is a potential mediator and marker of the tumor invasion of bladder cancer. Clin Cancer Res 2008;14(9): 2579–87.

23. Xu D, Suenaga N, Edelmann MJ, et al. Novel MMP-9 substrates in cancer cells revealed by a label-free quantitative proteomics approach. Mol Cell Proteomics 2008;7(11):2215–28.

24. Sardana G, Jung K, Stephan C, et al. Proteomic analysis of conditioned media from the PC3, LNCaP, and 22Rv1 prostate cancer cell lines: discovery and validation of candidate prostate cancer biomarkers. J Proteome Res 2008;7(8):3329–38.

25. Kulasingam V, Diamandis EP. Proteomics analysis of conditioned media from three breast cancer cell lines: a mine for biomarkers and therapeutic targets. Mol Cell Proteomics 2007;6(11):1997–2011.

26. Wu CC, Chen HC, Chen SJ, et al. Identification of collapsin response mediator protein-2 as a potential marker of colorectal carcinoma by comparative analysis of cancer cell secretomes. Proteomics 2008;8(2):316–32.

27. Goo YA, Liu AY, Ryu S, et al. Identification of secreted glycoproteins of human prostate and bladder stromal cells by comparative quantitative proteomics. Prostate 2009;69(1):49–61.

28. Mastrangelo L, Cassidy A, Mulholland F, et al. Serotonin receptors, novel targets of sulforaphane identified by proteomic analysis in Caco-2 cells. Cancer Res 2008;68(13):5487–91.

29. Mori-Iwamoto S, Kuramitsu Y, Ryozawa S, et al. Proteomics finding heat shock protein 27 as a biomarker for resistance of pancreatic cancer cells to gemcitabine. Int J Oncol 2007;31(6):1345–50.

30. Yang W, Hood BL, Chadwick SL, et al. Fatty acid synthase is up-regulated during hepatitis C virus infection and regulates hepatitis C virus entry and production. Hepatology 2008;48(5):1396–403.

31. Lemaitre G, Gonnet F, Vaigot P, et al. CD98, a novel marker of transient amplifying human keratinocytes. Proteomics 2005;5(14):3637–45.

32. Alldridge L, Metodieva G, Greenwood C, et al. Proteome profiling of breast tumors by gel electrophoresis and nanoscale electrospray ionization mass spectrometry. J Proteome Res 2008;7(4):1458–69.

33. Lu Q, Murugesan N, Macdonald JA, et al. Analysis of mouse brain microvascular endothelium using immuno-laser capture microdissection coupled to a hybrid linear ion trap with Fourier transform-mass spectrometry proteomics platform. Electrophoresis 2008;29(12):2689–95.

34. Hood BL, Darfler MM, Guiel TG, et al. Proteomic analysis of formalin-fixed prostate cancer tissue. Mol Cell Proteomics 2005;4(11):1741–53.

35. Hwang SI, Thumar J, Lundgren DH, et al. Direct cancer tissue proteomics: a method to identify candidate cancer biomarkers from formalin-fixed paraffin-embedded archival tissues. Oncogene 2007;26(1):65–76.

36. Patel V, Hood BL, Molinolo AA, et al. Proteomic analysis of laser-captured paraffin-embedded tissues: a molecular portrait of head and neck cancer progression. Clin Cancer Res 2008;14(4):1002–14.

37. Cheung W, Darfler MM, Alvarez H, et al. Application of a global proteomic approach to archival precursor lesions: deleted in malignant brain tumors 1 and tissue transglutaminase 2 are upregulated in pancreatic cancer precursors. Pancreatology 2008;8(6):608–16.

38. Caprioli RM, Farmer TB, Gile J. Molecular imaging of biological samples: localization of peptides and proteins using MALDI-TOF MS. Anal Chem 1997;69(23): 4751–60.

39. Lemaire R, Menguellet SA, Stauber J, et al. Specific MALDI imaging and profiling for biomarker hunting and validation: fragment of the 11S proteasome activator complex, Reg alpha fragment, is a new potential ovary cancer biomarker. J Proteome Res 2007;6(11):4127–34.
40. Chaurand P, Rahman MA, Hunt T, et al. Monitoring mouse prostate development by profiling and imaging mass spectrometry. Mol Cell Proteomics 2008;7(2):411–23.
41. Pieper R, Gatlin CL, Makusky AJ, et al. The human serum proteome: display of nearly 3700 chromatographically separated protein spots on two-dimensional electrophoresis gels and identification of 325 distinct proteins. Proteomics 2003;3(7):1345–64.
42. Issaq HJ, Xiao Z, Veemstra TD. Serum and plasma proteomics. Chem Rev 2007; 107(8):3601–20.
43. Tirumalai RS, Chan KC, Prieto DA, et al. Characterization of the low molecular weight human serum proteome. Mol Cell Proteomics 2003;2(10):1096–103.
44. Mehta A, Ross S, Lowenthal M, et al. Biomarker amplification by serum carrier protein binding. Dis Markers 2003–2004;19(1):1–10.
45. Zhou M, Lucas DA, Chan KC, et al. An investigation into the human serum "interactome". Electrophoresis 2004;25(9):1289–98.
46. Lowenthal MS, Mehta AI, Frogale K, et al. Analysis of albumin-associated peptides and proteins from ovarian cancer patients. Clin Chem 2005;51(10): 1933–45.
47. Faca VM, Song KS, Wang H, et al. A mouse to human search for plasma proteome changes associated with pancreatic tumor development. PLoS Med 2008;5(6):e123.
48. Sedlaczek P, Frydecka I, Gabrys M, et al. Comparative analysis of CA125, tissue polypeptide specific antigen, and soluble interleukin-2 receptor alpha levels in sera, cyst, and ascitic fluids from patients with ovarian carcinoma. Cancer 2002;95(9):1886–93.
49. Hu Y, Malone JP, Fagan AM, et al. Comparative proteomic analysis of intra- and interindividual variation in human cerebrospinal fluid. Mol Cell Proteomics 2005; 4(12):2000–9.
50. Waller LN, Shores K, Knapp DR. Shotgun proteomic analysis of cerebrospinal fluid using off-gel electrophoresis as the first-dimension separation. J Proteome Res 2008;7(10):4577–84.
51. Pan S, Zhu D, Quinn JF, et al. A combined dataset of human cerebrospinal fluid proteins identified by multi-dimensional chromatography and tandem mass spectrometry. Proteomics 2007;7(3):469–73.
52. Ranganathan S, Williams E, Ganchev P, et al. Proteomic profiling of cerebrospinal fluid identifies biomarkers for amyotrophic lateral sclerosis. J Neurochem 2005; 95(5):1461–71.
53. Choe L, D'Ascenzo M, Relkin NR, et al. 8-plex quantitation of changes in cerebrospinal fluid protein expression in subjects undergoing intravenous immunoglobulin treatment for Alzheimer's disease. Proteomics 2007;7(20):3651–60.
54. Klein PM, Lawrence JA. Lavage and nipple aspiration of breast ductal fluids: a source of biomarkers for environmental mutagenesis. Environ Mol Mutagen 2002;39(2–3):127–33.
55. Varnum SM, Covington CC, Woodbury RL, et al. Proteomic characterization of nipple aspirate fluid: identification of potential biomarkers of breast cancer. Breast Cancer Res Treat 2003;80(1):87–97.
56. Shaw JL, Smith CR, Diamandis EP. Proteomic analysis of human cervico-vaginal fluid. J Proteome Res 2007;6(7):2859–65.

57. Gortzak-Uzan L, Ignatchenko A, Evangelou AI, et al. A proteome resource of ovarian cancer ascites: integrated proteomic and bioinformatic analyses to identify putative biomarkers. J Proteome Res 2008;7(1):339–51.

58. Celis JE, Gromov P, Cabezon T, et al. Proteomic characterization of the interstitial fluid perfusing the breast tumor microenvironment: a novel resource for biomarker and therapeutic target discovery. Mol Cell Proteomics 2004;3(4): 327–44.

59. Huang CM, Ananthaswamy HN, Barnes S, et al. Mass spectrometric proteomics profiles of in vivo tumor secretomes: capillary ultrafiltration sampling of regressive tumor masses. Proteomics 2006;6(22):6107–16.

60. Kool J, Reubsaet L, Wesseldijk F, et al. Suction blister fluid as potential body fluid for biomarker proteins. Proteomics 2007;7(20):3638–50.

61. Chace DH. Mass spectrometry in the clinical laboratory. Chem Rev 2001;101(2): 445–77.

62. Chace DH. Mass spectrometry-based diagnostics: the upcoming revolution in disease detection has already arrived. Clin Chem 2003;49(7):1227–8, author reply 28–9.

63. Barr JR, Maggio VL, Patterson DG Jr, et al. Isotope dilution—mass spectrometric quantification of specific proteins: model application with apolipoprotein A-I. Clin Chem 1996;42(10):1676–82.

64. Barnidge DR, Dratz EA, Martin T, et al. Absolute quantification of the G protein-coupled receptor rhodopsin by LC/MS/MS using proteolysis product peptides and synthetic peptide standards. Anal Chem 2003;75(3):445–51.

65. Gerber SA, Rush J, Stemman O, et al. Absolute quantification of proteins and phosphoproteins from cell lysates by tandem MS. Proc Natl Acad Sci USA 2003;100(12):6940–5.

66. Abbatiello SE, Pan Y-X, Zhou M, et al. Mass spectrometric quantification of asparagine synthetase in circulating leukemia cells from acute lymphoblastic leukemia patients. J Proteomics 2008;71:61–70.

67. Appel IM, den Boer ML, Meijerink JP, et al. Up-regulation of asparagine synthetase expression is not linked to the clinical response L-asparaginase in pediatric acute lymphoblastic leukemia. Blood 2006;107(11):4244–9.

68. Su N, Pan YX, Zhou M, et al. Correlation between asparaginase sensitivity and asparagine synthetase protein content, but not mRNA, in acute lymphoblastic leukemia cell lines. Pediatr Blood Cancer 2008;50(2):274–9.

69. Ciustea M, Gutierrez JA, Abbatiello SE, et al. Efficient expression, purification, and characterization of C-terminally tagged, recombinant human asparagine synthetase. Arch Biochem Biophys 2005;440(1):18–27.

70. Villanueva J, Shaffer DR, Philip J, et al. Differential exoprotease activities confer tumor-specific serum peptidome patterns. J Clin Invest 2006;116(1):271–84.

71. Espina VA, Edmiston KH, Heiby M, et al. A portrait of tissue phosphoprotein stability in the clinical tissue procurement process. Mol Cell Proteomics 2008; 7(10):1998–2018.

Proteomics and Diabetic Retinopathy

Michael L. Merchant, PhD[a,b], Jon B. Klein, MD, PhD[b,c],*

KEYWORDS

- Proteomics • Diabetes • Mass spectrometry
- Electrophoresis • Retinopathy • Microvascular

Type-1 diabetes is a complex disease associated with an inability to control blood glucose levels, because of a hypoinsulinemic state resulting from a chronically low mass of insulin-producing pancreatic beta cells. The pervasive global increase in obesity, hyperlipidemia, and hypertension has now drawn equal attention to type-2 diabetes as also a disease influenced by problematic issues of perpetual insensitivity to circulating insulin levels and hypoinsulinemia.[1] The current estimates of the American Diabetes Association based on 2007 data suggest that there are 17.5 million diagnosed and 6.6 million undiagnosed diabetics (type-1 and type-2 diabetes) residing in the United States.[2] The most common microvascular complications of uncontrolled diabetes, diabetic nephropathy and diabetic retinopathy (DR), account for 29% and 15%, respectively, of the $116 billion expenditures associated with diabetes.[3] The Diabetes Complications and Control Trials reported for type-1 diabetes and the United Kingdom Prospective Diabetes Study reported for type-2 diabetes that onset and progression of these microvascular complications could be delayed or slowed through tight glucose control.[4–6] The combination of ill-defined etiology, numbers of affected individuals, and costs associated with disease progression, with the potential to slow or reverse some of the disease complications suggests that there is much to be gained from a greater understanding of the pathogenic mechanisms of diabetic microvascular disease. This article reviews the emerging role that proteomics has played in such an endeavor.

DR is a diabetic microvascular disease affecting the eyes.[6] DR can be staged as a complications gradient from mild nonproliferative retinopathy, moderate nonproliferative retinopathy, severe nonproliferative retinopathy, and proliferative retinopathy.[7] As with other complications of diabetes, DR may manifest as one of several clinical etiologies' including the swelling of retinal blood vessels with leakage of the contents

[a] Kidney Disease Program, University of Louisville, 615 South Preston Street, Louisville, KY 40202-1718, USA
[b] Clinical Proteomics Center, University of Louisville, Room 102S, Donald Baxter Research Building, 570 South Preston Street, Louisville, KY 40202, USA
[c] Veterans Affairs Medical Center, 800 Zorn Avenue, Louisville, KY 40206, USA
* Corresponding author. University of Louisville, Room 102S, Donald Baxter Research Building, 570 South Preston Street, Louisville, KY 40202.
E-mail address: jbklei01@gwise.louisville.edu (J.B. Klein).

Clin Lab Med 29 (2009) 139–149
doi:10.1016/j.cll.2009.01.008
0272-2712/09/$ – see front matter © 2009 Published by Elsevier Inc.

into the eyes or abnormal growth of blood vessels on the surface of the retinas. Current estimates suggest that for adults age 20 to 74 a total of 12,000 to 24,000 new cases of blindness resulting from these complications develop each year. Blindness or vision loss can be caused by proliferative DR (PDR), non-PDR, or diabetic macular edema. The most severe condition, PDR, is described by a proliferation of fragile blood vessels across the retina. The fragility of these blood vessels results in a loss of barrier integrity and leakage of blood into the eye causing a loss of vision. The potential exists within all stages of retinopathy and diabetic eye disease for leakage of fluid into the macula resulting in macular edema and a generalized blurring of vision.[8]

The proteomic method for scientific analysis is an approach rapidly to survey the proteome (complete inventory of proteins expressed within a biologic sample). With this method, biologic samples, such as lysates of retinal epithelial cells or vitreous fluid, are systematically analyzed with the intent of identifying, quantifying, and discerning the function of all observable proteins. The application of the proteomic method for comparison of disease and control samples allows for the rapid development of a hypothesis used to understand or explain aspects of disease biology, such as disease initiation, progression, or remission.[9] Many underlying methods used in proteomics have been used for decades, although recent proteomic advances have been driven by on-going developments in a set of core technologies including methods to separate complex mixtures of proteins[10] and peptides, soft ionization approaches used to characterize biologic molecules by mass spectrometry (MS),[11–13] and advanced computer-assisted data analyses approaches capable of handling complex data sets.[14] The insights gained from proteomic experiments should optimally allow for a better understanding of disease state initiation or propagation. Although proteomics is a relatively recent development for science, its limited application to the study of DR has already yielded impressive results.

APPLICATION OF PROTEOMICS TO THE STUDY OF ANIMAL MODELS OF DIABETIC RETINOPATHY

Murine models have developed into the principal model system for experimental studies of diabetic complications including DR, possibly because of the availability of both chemically induced diabetes with streptozotocin or alloxan and also the ability to develop unique genetic, sometimes spontaneous, models of diabetes.[15–17] Although most murine models have been shown to recapitulate some or many aspects of the known natural history of DR, no animal model perfectly matches human pathophysiology. Obrosova and colleagues[18] compared male Wistar rats and male C57 black 6/J mice as models of moderate- to high-dose streptozotocin-induced diabetes and selected DR-relevant end points to focus their studies on the early biochemical changes in murine retinas. They observed that in the short-term streptozotocin rat model, increased activity of the sorbitol pathway, increased oxidative stress as measured by levels of lipid peroxidation products, and glutathione concentrations heightened poly-ADP-ribose polymerase activation and altered reduction-oxidation status vis-à-vis NAD+/NADH ratios. The increase in sorbitol pathway intermediates, such as sorbitol and fructose, is an indication of enhanced activity of aldose reductase. Aldose reductase itself has been associated with increased vascular permeability and vascular endothelial growth factor overexpression and concomitant retinal neovascularization.[19] These alterations were muted or absent in the retinas of mice receiving high-dose streptozotocin. The well-known and strong mouse strain–dependent effect on response to streptozotocin toxicity suggests that these observations might be different in mouse strains other than the one tested.[17]

Recent proteomic studies on the neural retina of diabetic rats suggested the proteome to be complex and containing several thousand proteins and protein isoforms. Wang and colleagues[20] used high-resolution two-dimensional electrophoresis (2DE) with 24-cm isoelectric focusing strips in the first electrophoretic dimension to evaluate the retinal proteome of adult male Sprague-Dawley rats fed a high-fat diet and then given a 9-week series of low-dose (35 mg/kg body weight), intraperitoneal injections of freshly prepared streptozotocin. This model is suggested to recapitulate a type-2 diabetic state wherein the animals develop an obese and hyperlipidemic phenotype before a loss of insulin secretion resulting from streptozotocin administration. Weekly blood glucose measurements were used to follow the induction of diabetes. A blood glucose threshold value of 13.3 mmol/L or greater was used to distinguish the diabetic state and as the study inclusion criteria. Unfortunately, classical measures of diabetic renal damage, such as urine protein or urine albumin measurements, were not taken. These measures of diabetic renal microvascular disease could have values for use as a surrogate marker of diabetic retinal damage, allowing another measure of inclusion-exclusion into defining the study groups.[21] A total of 2702 ± 21 spots were observed across three gels of retinal samples from diabetic rats. In comparing diabetic and nondiabetic rats, a total of 150 protein spots were determined to be significantly different between the two groups. In these animals, 68 proteins were more abundant and 82 proteins were less abundant in the diabetic retinal proteomes. Using MS, 20 protein spots were identified and these included metabolic enzymes (glutamine synthetase, alpha enolase, glyceraldehyde-3-phosphate dehydrogenase, pyridoxal phosphate phosphatase, retinal dehydrogenase); chaperones and cochaperones (glucose-regulated protein 75, stress-induced phosphoprotein-1); proteases (leucine aminopeptidase-2); enzymes synthesizing nitric oxide synthetase antagonists (dimethylarginine dimethlyaminohydrolase-2); proteosomal proteins (proteosome alpha subunit); lipid and calcium binding proteins (lipocortin-1); protease inhibitors (serine proteinase inhibitor-clade B member 1b); and five isoforms of the retinal-specific protein alpha crystallin. The up-regulation of alpha crystallin was confirmed using immunoblot analysis. The increased abundance of retinal alpha crystallin in this type-2 diabetic model is consistent with data reported for retinal alpha crystallin expression in rat streptozotocin models of diabetes. Alpha crystallins are small heat shock proteins that among other functions participate in abrogating heat or oxidative stress-induced protein aggregation[22] and inhibiting apoptosis,[23] both important features of diabetic retinal disease.

In a similar study, Quin and colleagues[24] used a combination of 2DE and matrix-assisted laser desorption ionization (MALDI) time-of-flight (TOF) MS and liquid chromatography (LC)–coupled electrospray ionization (ESI) MS to compare the proteome of normal and diabetic rat retinas. An aspect of this work that distinguishes it from the work of Wang and colleagues[20] was the focus on the (single high-dose) streptozotocin-induced alteration of the retinal proteome following 10 weeks of hyperglycemia. The changes that were observed in these studies were hypothesized to mimic early alterations in the retinal proteome and are more comparable with the diabetic features involved with disease complication induction. A total of 168 proteins were identified, of which 35 proteins were differentially regulated by the diabetic state, 24 proteins were only visualized within the diabetic animal retinal gel images, and 37 proteins were absent from the diabetic animal retinal gel images. These striking observations should be considered to be a function of either unique posttranslational modifications of existing proteins, protein isoforms resulting from sample handling, or an intrinsic limitation of the sensitivity of the protein stain used to image the gels, rather than an absolution expressional induction or repression of more than one third of all observed proteins. The differentially regulated proteins included unique isoforms of cytoskeletal proteins (tubulin); metabolic enzymes (ATP synthase B subunit, glutamine synthase, pyridoxine kinase, enolase, pyruvate dehydrogenase, glutamine ammonia ligase, glyceraldehyde-3-phosphate dehydrogenase, fructose bisphosphate aldolase A, superoxide dismutase, tyrosine-3-monooxygenase); chaperones (chaperonin containing TCPI subunit, profilin 2); calcium and phospholipid binding proteins (calreticulin, calbindin 2); protease inhibitors (cystatin B); and retinal proteins (crystallin B2, phosducin chain C). Although many of these proteins were observed as distinctly different protein isoforms in the 2DE gels, some proteins were observed strongly up-regulated (heat shock proteins 70A and 8, aldehyde reductase 1, platelet-activating factor alpha 2, and beta catenin complex b) and strongly down-regulated (Reg-1 binding protein, apocellular retinoic acid binding protein B, dimethylarginine dimethoaminohydrolase, proteosome alpha 6 and alpha 1 subunits, aflatoxin aldehyde reductase, and dystrophin-related protein 2). Although some of these protein changes, such as dimethylarginine dimethlyaminohydrolases and proteosomal subunits, are consistent with those observed by Wang and colleagues,[20] other proteins beta catenin complex b and dystrophin-related protein 2 suggest that alterations of the retinal cell-cell junctions occur early in the diabetic state. This conclusion is consistent with an early loss of barrier integrity, development of retinal vascular permeability, and leakage of blood into the eye causing a loss of vision.

APPLICATION OF PROTEOMICS TO THE STUDY OF DIABETIC RETINOPATHY IN HUMANS

In comparison with other fields, such as cancer, the application of proteomics to the study of DR is a relatively recent event. Most of these studies have been devoted toward establishing retinal proteomes and proteome expression changes with disease. Most of the published studies used classical protein separation methods, such as one- and two-dimensional gel electrophoresis.

Garcia-Rameriez and colleagues[25] and Simo and colleagues[26] applied the technique of difference in gel electrophoresis (DIGE) to the study PDR and the vitreous proteome. DIGE is a 2DE method designed for higher throughput analyses of protein samples.[27] This is based on the ability to mix two samples, such as diabetic vitreous and control vitreous, and then coelectrophoreses the labeled proteins. The goal of this method is to reduce systematic variability associated with the 2DE method and to simplify the process of making between gel comparisons. The admixture of protein samples is easily differentiated in the gel because of the covalent modification of each protein sample with one of three cyanine dyes. The dyes are chemically reactive with the amino groups found on lysine side chains and the protein N-terminal α-amino groups. These dyes are commercially referred to as Cy-2, Cy-3, and Cy-5. Most frequently Cy-3 and Cy-5 dyes are used to label pairs of case and control protein samples. The Cy-2 dye is used to label a pooled protein sample derived from equivalent mass aliquots of all samples and used as an internal standard. The DIGE experiment involves mixing equal amounts of labeled protein and coelectrophoresing the single sample for the 2DE experiment. The gel is sequentially imaged using a fluorescence scanner using wavelengths specific to the Cy-2, -3, or -5 dyes. The fluorescence intensities of the individual spots or the entire gel for all Cy-3 or Cy-5 scans are normalized to the Cy-2 scans. The normalization to the pooled protein sample makes possible a direct comparison of protein spots matched by imaging software as the same protein spot but residing in separate gels. The control vitreous in these settings was from nondiabetic patients with macular holes. These studies both had carefully designed criteria for exclusion of patients including a history of diabetes or renal disease, and recent history of vitreous hemorrhage (<3 month) or photocoagulation (<6 month). Total protein was isolated from these vitreous samples and individual samples labeled with one of two cyanine-dyes (Cy-3 or Cy-5) and an internal standard made from a pool of all samples labeled with Cy-2 dye. Approximately 1400 spots were observed across all gels. A total of 41 proteins were determined to be significantly differentially abundant at a P value less than 0.05 considering a threshold diabetic to control protein expression ratio of 1.4. Twenty-eight proteins were up-regulated in the diabetic state and 13 proteins were down-regulated in the diabetic state. Eleven proteins were identified including eight up-regulated proteins (fibrinogen A, β_2 glycoprotein-1, complement factor B, zinc-alpha glycoprotein, complement C3, complement C9, complement C4-B, and apolipoprotein A-I) and three down-regulated proteins (inter-alpha trypsin inhibitor heavy chain 2, pigment-epithelium derived factor, and interphoton retinoid binding protein). Garcia-Rameriz and colleagues[25] used immunoblotting approaches in an expanded sample set to validate the DIGE findings successfully for three up-regulated (zinc alpha glycoprotein, complement C3, and complement factor B) and two down-regulated proteins (pigment-epithelium derived factor and interphoton retinoid binding protein). Garcia-Rameriz and colleagues[25] explored the source of these differences by quantifying the levels of these proteins in the patients' serum and the levels of the mRNA in the retina. Additional experiments determined that these differences were not observed in these same patients' serum and were specifically intravitreal. Using donor eyes from diabetics and nondiabetics, Garcia-Rameriz and colleagues[25] determined retinal mRNA levels for these five proteins. In each case the trend in protein expression and mRNA expression was coordinated. In two instances, complement C3 and interphoton retinoid binding protein, the differences in retinal mRNA expression was statistically significant. In an extension of the work of Garcia-Rameriz and colleagues,[25] Simo and colleagues[26] used DIGE to identify apolipoprotein H and confirmed apolipoprotein A-I as being increased in the vitreous of PDR patients. The proteomic findings were validation orthogonally with immunoblot and quantitative reverse-transcriptase polymerase chain reaction experiments using retinal mRNA. Although the finding of apolipoprotein H regulation is novel and suggests an inflammatory contribution to the mechanism of PDR progression, more work is necessary to build on this hypothesis.

The vitreous proteome has been demonstrated by electrophoresis to have moderate complexity as demonstrated by the number of observed protein spots on large format 2DE gels. In some regards, 2DE is a top-down proteomics approach in that proteins are separated and differences in protein expression are detected before selection for identification by MS-based methods. A complementary method is the bottom-up approach to proteomic analysis. With this approach a proteome is first digested with a protease, such as trypsin, chymotrypsin, or an aspartic acid protease. This peptide mixture is then fractionated using one- or two-dimensional LC and interrogated indirectly (eg, with LC-MALDI-TOF MS-MS) or directly (eg, with LC-ESI-MS-MS). The successfully identified peptides are used to reconstruct the sample proteome. These approaches, especially the LC-ESI MS-MS method, enable the identification of hundreds to a few thousand proteins with single samples.

Kim and colleagues[28] used a battery of proteomic tools to study and compile an inventory of the vitreous proteomes of nondiabetic patients and patients with PDR. Initial proteomics work was directed at increasing the sensitivity of the 2DE analysis by first fractionating the samples using antibody-based affinity chromatography columns to immunodeplete the 12 most abundant serum proteins from the vitreous samples. Two general assumptions of the antibody-based approach of abundant protein depletion from the target sample are first that few or no proteins codepleted with the targeted proteins and second there is an overall increase in the sensitivity to detect low-abundant proteins. Unfortunately, in this case Kim and colleagues[28] determined that more proteins were nonspecifically depleted from the vitreous sample than were expected to be specifically depleted. It was also shown that the overall increase in sensitivity using the 2DE approach was not significant. The vitreous samples were reanalyzed using an approach to immuno-deplete albumin and Ig followed by analysis of the lower-abundant proteins by a LC-MAL-DI-TOF MS-MS method and a nano-flow LC-ESI MS-MS method. An aggregate database of vitreous proteins was established from the 2DE, LC-MALDI-TOF MS-MS, and nano-flow LC-ESI MS-MS data sets. A total of 531 proteins were identified, of which 230 had not previously been reported for the vitreous proteome. Although these studies did not identify a previously known PDR regulator, vascular endothelial growth factor,[29] the protein carbonic anhydrase-I (CA-I) was detected as a proteome component. A significant work by Gao and colleagues,[30] discussed later, identifies mechanistically the role of CA-I in the progression of retinal vascular permeability.

Many proteomic studies of diabetic eye disease have focused on the study of differences between the vitreous proteomes of diabetics with and without proliferative retinopathy. Decanini and colleagues[31] instead applied a classical proteomics approach, 2DE, to the study of the retinal pigment epithelium proteome to understand better the changes that occur with early diabetes. Here, these studies involved donor eyes for microdissection and collection of the epithelium. As such, the fundus of each eye could be extensively evaluated for signs of PDR, microaneurysms, dot blot hemorrhages, or signs of hard exudation. Digital images were taken before and following removal of the neural retina and the retinal pigment epitheliums examined by two ophthalmologists. Exclusion criteria for this study included clinical evidence of retinal pathology and post-mortem changes in the retinal vasculature. Inclusion criteria for the diabetic group included past medical history of diabetes but no evidence of retinal pathology. Proteins from early diabetic patients without retinal pathology were separated using 2DE, and proteins were imaged after staining with a highly sensitive fluorescent protein dye (Flamingo fluorescent stain; Bio-Rad, Hercules, California). Following image quantification, a total of 325 protein spots were imaged. Although 31 of the 325 spots were significantly differentially abundant between the two groups, only 18 proteins spots were successfully identified; of these 18 spots, 15 proteins were up-regulated and 3 were down-regulated with diabetes. The proteins up-regulated with diabetes included metabolic enzymes (aldehyde dehydrogenase, dihydrolipoyl dehydrogenase); structural proteins (actin); lipid and calcium binding proteins (annexins A4 and A7); proteases (cathepsin D); transport proteins (retinaldehyde binding protein, selenium binding protein 1, sterol carrier protein X); and molecular chaperones (elongation factor 2, glucose regulated protein 75, heat shock protein 71, protein disulfide isomerase A3). The proteins down-regulated with diabetes included metabolic enzymes gamma enolase, phosphoglycerate mutase 1, and succinyl coenzyme A: 3-ketoacid coenzyme A. Although the strongest expressional change was observed with a fivefold increase in actin with the diabetic state, perhaps the most striking change was in the numbers of mitochondrial proteins whose expression was increased by 35% to 105%. This observation is consistent with the association of the molecular genesis of diabetic pathology with dysregulation of mitochondrial biology.[32]

TARGETED PROTEOMIC STUDIES AND IMMUNOPROTEOMIC ANALYSIS OF THE VITREOUS PROTEOME USING DIABETIC SERA

Data exist to suggest that circulating autoantibodies to retinal proteins contribute to retina destruction in patients with DR. Anh and colleagues[33] conducted a targeted immunoproteomics study using undepleted patient sera first to evaluate immunoglobulin cross-reactivity to retinal cytosolic proteins and second to identify putative immunogenic proteins. The study compared the sera of four groups of nonhypertensive patients including controls, diabetics without retinopathy, diabetics with DR, and diabetics with PDR, for the ability to cross-react with retinal proteins isolated from normal human retinal tissue. The hypothesis was first addressed using 1DE and 2DE to separate retinal membrane and cytosolic proteins, respectively, followed by transfer of the resolved proteins onto nitrocellulose membranes. The patients' sera were used as the primary antibody solutions and the total immunogenicity of the sera was evaluated following horseradish-linked secondary antibody and image development on film. A large number of weak immunopositive bands were observed in membrane protein preparations with all sera and with cytosolic protein preparations using normal patient sera. Compared with controls' sera all diabetic sera produced more intense staining in cytosolic protein immunoblots experiments. The diversity of immunopositive bands and the intensity of staining correlated with severity of DR. A total of 29 proteins were selected for further study and 20 proteins corresponding to 18 gene products were identified using LC-ESI MS-MS. Most identified proteins were observed in diabetics with DR and diabetics with PDR and fewer were observed in diabetics with retinopathy and normals. Four protein spots identified as creatine kinase B, aldolase C, phosphoglycerate kinase 1, and carbonic anhydrase II were observed in diabetics with DR and also PDR but not control diabetics or normals. Aldolase C, previously known as a "brain-specific protein," was selected for further study using ELISA. The results of these experiments demonstrated increased levels of aldolase C immunoreactivity in the sera of diabetic patients without DR compared with normals and moreover increased aldolase C immunoreactivity in the sera of diabetic patients with DR or PDR over diabetics without DR. Interestingly, there was no significant difference in the levels of immunogenicity observed in the sera of diabetics with DR as compared with diabetics with PDR.

PROTEOMIC DISCOVERY EXPERIMENTS OF THE DIABETIC VITREOUS LEADS TO A BETTER MECHANISTIC UNDERSTANDING OF DISEASE PROGRESSION

Large-scale proteomic experiments are often able to produce a robust inventory of abundantly expressed proteins, which is often the desired experimental end point. A comparative analysis of these protein lists can then be used to derive a protein knowledge base and develop testable hypotheses. From the perspective of clinical proteomics, it is most advantageous and desirable if those experiments also lead toward a more concrete understanding of disease mechanisms, whether it is disease initiation or disease progression. Recently, such proteomic experiments have been conducted and used to advance the understanding of the vitreous proteome and how changes in that proteome can contribute to diabetic microvascular disease pathogenesis.

Gao and colleagues[30] used a combination of classical proteomic experiments (1DE with MS-based protein identification) and recently developed methods of label-free MS-based, semiquantitative spectral counting approaches to study the vitreous proteome of diabetic patients. The study was conducted using undiluted vitreous samples obtained from 25 subjects (nondiabetic; diabetic without DR [non-PDR]; diabetic with DR). A randomized subgroup of patient samples was selected for proteomic discovery experiments based on 1DE and LC-MS to characterize the vitreous proteome. An expanded set of vitreous samples was used for validation experiments by immunoblot. The vitreous proteomes of nondiabetic, non-PDR, and PDR patients were not complex, hence, application of 1DE was not limiting to the study. A total of 64, 113, and 107 proteins were identified, respectively, with significant overlap between the three groups. The qualitative differences in protein expression (or abundance) between the three groups were estimated using the MS-MS data. The approaches used included the direct comparison between differences in identified proteins (presence to absence analysis) and the extent of peptide coverage for proteins overlapping between groups. A semiquantitative label-free method known as "spectral counting" was analyzed by a statistical method. An assumption of the spectral counting method is that the numbers of unique peptides assigned to a protein are linearly related to the protein abundance. The numbers of unique peptides for each protein were compared between groups by a Kruskal-Wallis analysis to assign a measure of statistical difference for protein abundance. Thirty-one proteins were determined to be significantly different with this analysis. These proteins could be functionally assigned by gene ontology analysis into groups including transport proteins, acute-phase proteins, proteins involved in cell growth, maintenance and metabolism, complement systems proteins, and cell adhesion proteins.

A series of immunoblot-based validation experiments suggested the protein with the strongest-fold expression increase comparing nondiabetic with non-PDR (greater than eightfold; $P<.05$) or with PDR (greater than 15-fold; $P<.01$) was extracellular carbonic anhydrase I (CA-I); similar results were also observed in individuals with quiescent PDR and non-PDR. Other proteins demonstrating increased abundance in PDR by immunoblotting experiments were carbonic anhydrase-II, angiotensinogen, complement-I inhibitor, and pigmented epithelium-derived factor. CA-I was correlated positively by a Spearman correlation analysis to the presence of 14 other proteins including plasma proteins and erythrocyte proteins, suggesting CA-I's vitreous presence resulted form ocular hemorrhage. Although CA-I had not been previously associated with retinal vascular permeability, an inhibitor of CA activity, acetazolamide, had been previously reported to be beneficial for patients with diabetic macular edema. These data and the disparity of extracellular CA-I in PDR vitreous compared with other vitreous sample groups formed the basis for pursuing additional experiments to understand better CA-I's potential role in disease pathogenesis.

Gao and colleagues[30] elegantly demonstrated using diabetic rat models an association of retinal vascular permeability with intravitreal injection of the vitreous of diabetics with proliferative retinopathy and also with intravitreal injection of CA-I. The permeability was reduced with coinjection of acetazolamide. The magnitude of retinal vascular permeability was greater than that produced by intravitreal injection of vascular endothelial growth factor, a substance considered to the principle factor responsible for retinal vascular permeability in both PDR and diabetic macular edema. Interestingly, the extent of retinal vascular permeability was increased proportionally with intravitreal injection of both CA-I and vascular endothelial growth factor. Additional experiments demonstrated an association of CA-I enzymatic activity with an increase in ocular pH, with increased retinal thickness, and with increased outer nuclear layer thickness.

Using a proteomics approach, Gao and colleagues[30] evaluated the effects of intravitreal coinjection of CA-I with proteins positively correlating with CA-I, including the protein C1-INH, an inhibitor of serpins (serine proteases). C1-INH deficiency had previously been associated with increases in vascular permeability increased bradykinin production and activation of the bradykinin-2 receptor. Coinjection of C1-INH with CA-I inhibited CA-I–induced retinal vascular permeability but not vascular endothelial growth factor–induced retinal vascular permeability. Gao and colleagues[30] used additional experiments to demonstrate the involvement of both the bradykinin-1 and bradykinin-2 receptors, and the proteolytic activity kallikrein are required for CA-I induction of retinal vascular permeability. These experiments and additional experiments using antagonists of downstream targets of bradykinin receptor activation demonstrated a role for the kallikrein-kinin system in promoting retinal vascular permeability following intraocular hemorrhage. A significant result of this work is the delineation of a mechanistic pathway involved in disease progression. The knowledge of the vitreous proteome (more recently updated by Gao and colleagues)[34] and the elucidated pathway provides for the rational design of experiments used to intervene in the incremental steps necessary for disease progression.

SUMMARY

Despite significant research on many fronts, the global diabetes pandemic and its attendant complications, such as DR, remains complex and poorly understood. Proteomic approaches have been used to deal with these complexities through methods to increase the fractional abundance of low-abundant proteins, methods directly to compare protein samples either using chemical labeling methods, such as DIGE, or label-free methods, such as that of Gao and colleagues, to identify and comparatively analyze proteins directly in the MS. It is more likely that a single protein does not initiate disease progression but rather multiple vitreous-resident serum proteins like apolipoprotein A-I and apolipoprotein H or CA-I and C1-INH will likely contribute to the pathogenic mechanisms, such as those demonstrated here leading to retinal vascular bed permeability and progression of PDR. Substantial work remains to understand better the initiation and progression of non-PDR, PDR, and diabetic macular edema in the context of why some type-1 diabetics and why many type-2 diabetics do not progress toward loss of vision and blindness.

REFERENCES

1. Gavin JR III. Diagnosis and classification of diabetes mellitus. Diabetes Care 2006; 29(Suppl 1):S43–8.
2. American Diabetes Association. Economic costs of diabetes in the U.S. in 2007. Diabetes Care 2008;31:596–615.
3. UK Prospective Diabetes Study Group. Tight blood pressure control and risk of macrovascular and microvascular complications in type 2 diabetes: UKPDS 38. UK Prospective Diabetes Study Group. BMJ 1998;317:703–13.
4. The Diabetes Control and Complications Trial Research Group. The effect of intensive treatment of diabetes on the development and progression of long-term complications in insulin-dependent diabetes mellitus. The Diabetes Control and Complications Trial Research Group. N Engl J Med 1993;329:977–86.
5. Girach A, Manner D, Porta M. Diabetic microvascular complications: can patients at risk be identified? A review. Int J Clin Pract 2006;60:1471–83.
6. Kohner EM. Microvascular disease: what does the UKPDS tell us about diabetic retinopathy? Diabet Med 2008;25(Suppl 2):20–4.
7. Williams R, Airey M, Baxter H, et al. Epidemiology of diabetic retinopathy and macular oedema: a systematic review. Eye 2004;18:963–83.
8. Fong DS, Aiello L, Gardner TW, et al. Retinopathy in diabetes. Diabetes Care 2004;27(Suppl 1):S84–7.
9. Merchant ML, Klein JB. Proteomics and diabetic nephropathy. Semin Nephrol 2007;27:627–36.
10. Issaq H, Veenstra T. Two-dimensional polyacrylamide gel electrophoresis (2D-PAGE): advances and perspectives. Biotechniques 2008;44:697–8, 700.
11. Zhou M, Veenstra T. Mass spectrometry: m/z 1983-2008. Biotechniques 2008;44: 667–8, 670.

12. Matt P, Fu Z, Fu Q, et al. Biomarker discovery: proteome fractionation and separation in biological samples. Physiol Genomics 2008;33:12–7.
13. Qian WJ, Jacobs JM, Liu T, et al. Advances and challenges in liquid chromatography-mass spectrometry-based proteomics profiling for clinical applications. Mol Cell Proteomics 2006;5:1727–44.
14. Chalkley RJ, Hansen KC, Baldwin MA. Bioinformatic methods to exploit mass spectrometric data for proteomic applications. Meth Enzymol 2005;402:289–312.
15. Tesch GH, Allen TJ. Rodent models of streptozotocin-induced diabetic nephropathy. Nephrology (Carlton) 2007;12:261–6.
16. Rees DA, Alcolado JC. Animal models of diabetes mellitus. Diabet Med 2005;22: 359–70.
17. Breyer MD, Bottinger E, Brosius FC III, et al. Mouse models of diabetic nephropathy. J Am Soc Nephrol 2005;16:27–45.
18. Obrosova IG, Drel VR, Kumagai AK, et al. Early diabetes-induced biochemical changes in the retina: comparison of rat and mouse models. Diabetologia 2006;49:2525–33.
19. Kato N, Yashima S, Suzuki T, et al. Long-term treatment with fidarestat suppresses the development of diabetic retinopathy in STZ-induced diabetic rats. J Diabet Complications 2003;17:374–9.
20. Wang YD, Wu JD, Jiang ZL, et al. Comparative proteome analysis of neural retinas from type 2 diabetic rats by two-dimensional electrophoresis. Curr Eye Res 2007;32:891–901.
21. Arar NH, Freedman BI, Adler SG, et al. Heritability of the severity of diabetic retinopathy: the FIND-Eye study. Invest Ophthalmol Vis Sci 2008;49:3839–45.
22. Horwitz J. Alpha-crystallin can function as a molecular chaperone. Proc Natl Acad Sci U S A 1992;89:10449–53.
23. Kamradt MC, Chen F, Cryns VL. The small heat shock protein alpha B-crystallin negatively regulates cytochrome c- and caspase-8-dependent activation of caspase-3 by inhibiting its autoproteolytic maturation. J Biol Chem 2001;276: 16059–63.
24. Quin GG, Len AC, Billson FA, et al. Proteome map of normal rat retina and comparison with the proteome of diabetic rat retina: new insight in the pathogenesis of diabetic retinopathy. Proteomics 2007;7:2636–50.
25. Garcia-Ramirez M, Canals F, Hernandez C, et al. Proteomic analysis of human vitreous fluid by fluorescence-based difference gel electrophoresis (DIGE): a new strategy for identifying potential candidates in the pathogenesis of proliferative diabetic retinopathy. Diabetologia 2007;50:1294–303.
26. Simo R, Higuera M, Garcia-Ramirez M, et al. Elevation of apolipoprotein A-I and apolipoprotein H levels in the vitreous fluid and overexpression in the retina of diabetic patients. Arch Ophthalmol 2008;126:1076–81.
27. Timms JF, Cramer R. Difference gel electrophoresis. Proteomics 2008;8:4886–97.
28. Kim T, Kim SJ, Kim K, et al. Profiling of vitreous proteomes from proliferative diabetic retinopathy and nondiabetic patients. Proteomics 2007;7:4203–15.
29. Wirostko B, Wong TY, Simo R. Vascular endothelial growth factor and diabetic complications. Prog Retin Eye Res 2008;27:608–21.
30. Gao BB, Clermont A, Rook S, et al. Extracellular carbonic anhydrase mediates hemorrhagic retinal and cerebral vascular permeability through prekallikrein activation. Nat Med 2007;13:181–8.
31. Decanini A, Karunadharma PR, Nordgaard CL, et al. Human retinal pigment epithelium proteome changes in early diabetes. Diabetologia 2008;51:1051–61.

32. Patti ME. Gene expression in humans with diabetes and prediabetes: what have we learned about diabetes pathophysiology? Curr Opin Clin Nutr Metab Care 2004;7:383–90.

33. Ahn BY, Song ES, Cho YJ, et al. Identification of an anti-aldolase autoantibody as a diagnostic marker for diabetic retinopathy by immunoproteomic analysis. Proteomics 2006;6:1200–9.

34. Gao BB, Chen X, Timothy N, et al. Characterization of the vitreous proteome in diabetes without diabetic retinopathy and diabetes with proliferative diabetic retinopathy. J Proteome Res 2008;7:2516–25.

Index

Note: Page numbers of article titles are in **boldface** type.

A

ABI Q-star, 57
Abuminome, in cardiovascular disease, 87–88
Actin, in diabetic retinopathy, 142
Affinity-based enrichment, in autoantibody profiling, 31
Aldolase, in diabetic retinopathy, 143
Alzheimer's disease, biomarkers for, 127
Amyotrophic lateral sclerosis, biomarkers for, 127
Annexins, antibodies to, in lung cancer, 36–37
Antibody-lectin sandwich microarrays, 21–25
Anticoagulants, for cardiovascular proteomics, 89
Apolipoproteins, in diabetic retinopathy, 141
AQUA method, 105, 131
Ascites fluid, biomarkers in, 128
Asparagine synthetase, in leukemia, 131–132
Autoantibody profiling, for cancer detection, **29–44**
　　lung, 33–39
　　tumor antigens and, 30–33

B

Bacteria, antibodies to, glycoproteomics in, 18
Beckman Biomek system, 59
Biomarkers
　　for cancer, **113–136**
　　　　in saliva, **69–83**
　　　　instability of, in tissue, 4
　　　　ovarian, **45–53**
　　for cardiovascular disease, **85–97**
　　in formalin-fixed paraffin-embedded tissues, **99–111**
　　mass spectrometry patterns of. *See* Mass spectrometry, in biomarker discovery.
Biomek system, 59
Bladder cancer, biomarkers for, 120–121
Blister fluid, sampling of, 129
BMI-1 protein, antibodies to, in lung cancer, 34–35
Bradykinin, in diabetic retinopathy, 144–145
Brain cancer, biomarkers for, 121–122
Breast cancer
　　autoantibodies in, 34
　　biomarkers for, 120–121
　　　　in nipple aspirate, 128

Clin Lab Med 29 (2009) 151–158
doi:10.1016/S0272-2712(09)00023-7
0272-2712/09/$ – see front matter © 2009 Elsevier Inc. All rights reserved.

labmed.theclinics.com

Moving?

Make sure your subscription moves with you!

To notify us of your new address, find your **Clinics Account Number** (located on your mailing label above your name), and contact customer service at:

E-mail: elspcs@elsevier.com

800-654-2452 (subscribers in the U.S. & Canada)
314-453-7041 (subscribers outside of the U.S. & Canada)

Fax number: 314-523-5170

Elsevier Periodicals Customer Service
11830 Westline Industrial Drive
St. Louis, MO 63146

*To ensure uninterrupted delivery of your subscription, please notify us at least 4 weeks in advance of move.